DATE DUE

Integrative Treatment of Anxiety Disorders

Integrative Treatment of Anxiety Disorders

Edited by
James M. Ellison, M.D., M.P.H.

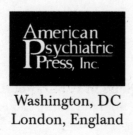

American Psychiatric Press, Inc.

Washington, DC
London, England

Copyright © 1996 American Psychiatric Press, Inc.
ALL RIGHTS RESERVED
Manufactured in the United States of America on acid-free paper
99 98 97 96   4 3 2 1
First Edition

American Psychiatric Press, Inc.
1400 K Street, N.W., Washington, DC   20005

Library of Congress Cataloging-in-Publication Data
Integrative treatment of anxiety disorders / edited by James M. Ellison.
    p.   cm.
    Includes bibliographical references and index.
    ISBN 0-88048-715-1
    1. Anxiety—Treatment.   I.   Ellison, James M., 1952-   .
    [DNLM: 1. Anxiety Disorders—drug therapy. 2. Psychotherapy. 3. Combined Modality Therapy.   WM 172 I603 1996]
    RC531.I56   1996
    616.85′22306—dc20
    DNLM/DLC   95-21836
    for Library of Congress   CIP

British Library Cataloguing in Publication Data
A CIP record is available from the British Library.

Contents

Contributors

Henry David Abraham, M.D.
Director of Substance Abuse Programs, New England Medical Center, Boston, Massachusetts; Clinical Professor of Psychiatry, Tufts University School of Medicine, Boston, Massachusetts

Nancy Bridges, L.I.C.S.W.
Clinical Supervisor, Department of Psychiatry, The Cambridge Hospital, Cambridge, Massachusetts; Lecturer on Psychiatry, Harvard Medical School, Boston, Massachusetts; Clinical Assistant Professor, Smith College School for Social Work, Northampton, Massachusetts

James M. Ellison, M.D., M.P.H.
Chief, Mental Health Department, Robert H. Ebert Burlington Health Center, Harvard Pilgrim Health Care, Burlington, Massachusetts; Consulting Psychiatrist, The Cambridge Hospital, Cambridge, Massachusetts; Associate Clinical Professor of Psychiatry, Harvard Medical School, Boston, Massachusetts; Lecturer, Department of Psychiatry, Tufts University School of Medicine, Boston, Massachusetts

Douglas H. Hughes, M.D.
Director, Psychiatric Emergency Services, The Cambridge Hospital, Cambridge, Massachusetts; Lecturer on Psychiatry, Harvard Medical School, Boston, Massachusetts

Satori Iwamoto, M.D., Ph.D.
Senior Fellow, Department of Medicine/Dermatology, University of Washington Medical Center, Seattle, Washington

R. Harris G. McCarter, Ph.D.
Staff Psychologist, Behavioral Medicine, The Cambridge Hospital, Cambridge, Massachusetts; Co-Director, Cambridge Associates in Psychotherapy and Mediation, Cambridge, Massachusetts; Instructor in Psychology, Department of Psychiatry, Harvard Medical School, Boston, Massachusetts

Christine Pfaelzer, M.D., M.P.H.
Resident in Psychiatry, New York State Psychiatric Institute of Columbia University, New York, New York

Sabrina M. Popp, M.D.
Staff Psychiatrist, Substance Abuse Treatment Program, Veterans Administration Hospital, Jamaica Plain, Massachusetts; Assistant Professor of Psychiatry, Tufts University School of Medicine, Boston, Massachusetts

Pamela Reeves, M.D.
Director of Somatic Therapies in Psychiatry, The Cambridge Hospital, Cambridge, Massachusetts; Instructor in Psychiatry, Harvard Medical School, Boston, Massachusetts

Brian F. Sands, M.D.
Director of Psychopharmacology, Substance Abuse Treatment Programs, Department of Veteran's Affairs Outpatient Clinic, Boston, Massachusetts; Assistant Professor, Department of Psychiatry, Tufts University School of Medicine, Boston, Massachusetts; Clinical Instructor, Department of Psychiatry, Harvard Medical School, Boston, Massachusetts

Allen Sherman, Ph.D.
Clinical Director, Behavioral Medicine Program, Arkansas Cancer Research Center, and Assistant Professor in Otolaryngology, University of Arkansas Medical Sciences, Little Rock, Arkansas

Robert G. Ziegler, M.D.
Co-Director, Child and Adolescent Outpatient Services, The Cambridge Hospital, Cambridge, Massachusetts; Clinical Director, Boundaries Therapy Center, Acton, Massachusetts; Instructor in Psychiatry, Harvard Medical School, Boston, Massachusetts; Staff Psychiatrist, Somerville Mental Health Center Child Service, Somerville, Massachusetts

Preface

A clash of doctrines is not a disaster—it is an opportunity.

Alfred North Whitehead

Driven by pressures both clinical and economic, we mental health clinicians have entered a new era of treatment integration. We increasingly find ourselves offering patients a mix of psychotherapy and pharmacotherapy in our efforts to improve treatment response. The clinical pressure for such integration arises because research has demonstrated impressive effects of either psychosocial or pharmacological interventions on a variety of patients' conditions. In particular, cognitive-behavior therapies have dramatically relieved mood and anxiety symptoms traditionally considered to require medication. At the same time, new and highly effective pharmacotherapies have been developed to address the morbidity of these disorders. These medications' effects often extend beyond mere symptom relief into the realm of new learning and personality change. As clinical experience and outcome data accumulate, they undermine too sharp a distinction between mind and brain. They also compel clinicians to be knowledgeable about the variety of treatments available for a given disorder so that they can help their patients to participate in an informed consent process regarding treatment options.

The economic pressures encouraging integrative treatment arise from the increasingly pervasive presence of managed care procedures. For better or worse, management of limited treatment resources is with us for the foreseeable future, forcing us to allocate our work as efficiently as possible. As we seek ways to enhance and accelerate our patients' progress, integrative treatment has become increasingly accepted. Particularly in the treatment of anxiety disorders, it appears that concurrent psychotherapy and pharmacotherapy may offer patients a greater breadth of relief, a quicker route to improvement, and perhaps a way of maintaining their gains over a more prolonged period of time.

In attempting to understand the syndromes of anxiety disorders, an appreciation of the interplay between psychotherapeutic and pharmacological treatments is particularly illuminating. Each modality directly affects the action of the other, resulting in a synergistic effect in many patients. In treating an agoraphobic individual with pharmacotherapy, for example, medication use may become the essential first step that allows the patient to leave home in order to participate in other treatment approaches. The simple alleviation of symptoms, however, is only part of what pharmacotherapy can accomplish. Panic disorder patients who receive appropriate pharmacotherapy often gain insight into the previously unsuspected extent of their disability. As the panic attacks become less frequent, such patients often realize how greatly they had been impaired by limited symptom attacks, anticipatory anxiety, performance anxiety, and other phenomena often seen in this disorder. In patients with obsessive-compulsive disorder (OCD), the appropriate use of medications often enhances psychotherapy by ushering a patient into new areas of insight. Very often, care providers will see a medication-responsive patient discover that his or her "disorder" has extended far into regions accepted as "personality." "Characteristic" behaviors ranging from circumscribed phenomena such as mental rituals, nail biting, or trichotillomania to very complex syndromes such as some forms of pathological jealousy, paraphilias, or apparent psychosis may respond impressively to medication treatment.

Psychotherapy, too, can powerfully affect symptoms often considered "biological." The most thoroughly investigated psychotherapeutic treatments of anxiety disorders fall within the realm of cognitive-behavioral approaches. Studies of cognitive-behavioral treatment of panic disorder patients, for example, have made it clear that panic attacks can be diminished through psychotherapy provided alone or adjunctively. Indeed, cognitive-behavioral psychotherapy has even been shown to prevent panic attacks induced chemically by means of an intravenous lactate infusion. Medication tapering can be facilitated, moreover, and relapse rates diminished in panic disorder patients who receive cognitive-behavior therapy as a component of their treatment.

The anxiety disorders are among the most frequently diagnosed mental disorders and account for much of our professional mental health activity. Although they contribute extensively to morbidity and dysfunction, these disorders are on the whole very responsive to treatment. This book reviews the anxiety disorders and their treatment alternatives, with particular emphasis on the integration of pharmacotherapy with cognitive-behavioral psychotherapy. Truly integrative treatment, in the authors' conception, consists of the orchestrated use of multiple treatment approaches, each of which has been shown effective and able to work synergistically. Some clinicians are single-handedly able to offer a variety of treatment modalities, but integrative treatment usually implies a collaborative effort among two or more clinicians. Issues of referral management, treatment planning, and collaboration are consequently also addressed in the chapters that follow. Because anxiety disorders are increasingly recognized in the pediatric, medically ill, and substance abusing populations, additional chapters address concerns more specific to those patient groups.

Integrative Treatment of Anxiety Disorders emerged from the enthusiasm generated by a Continuing Medical Education conference of the same name sponsored by The Cambridge Hospital. My collaborators and I, therefore, gratefully acknowledge the encouragement of Judith Platt, Ed.D, Malkah Notman, M.D., Deborah Moran, M.D., and our other Cambridge Hospital colleagues. We also acknowledge the contribution of the patients whose stories—disguised to protect anonymity—illustrate the principles of this book. I am indebted to The Cambridge Hospital's outstanding psychiatric residents for their continuing intellectual curiosity and their insightful discussions of the topics covered in this volume. My Harvard Community Health Plan colleagues Ginger Phakos, L.I.C.S.W., and Patricia DeLuca, R.N., C.S., deserve thanks for the valuable comments they offered on chapters in progress. Finally, my wife, Patricia Harney, has provided the space in our lives for the completion of this project and has encouraged its progress at every stage. She has more than earned my gratitude through her generous love and perceptive contributions.

James M. Ellison, M.D., M.P.H.

Generalized Anxiety Disorder, Social Phobia, and Performance Anxiety: Pharmacotherapy and Aspects of Integration With Psychotherapy

Brian F. Sands, M.D.

I n this chapter I discuss the medications currently available for treatment of several anxiety disorders and provide guidelines for integrating their use with psychotherapy. The topic is broad because anxiety, a nonspecific symptom, reaches beyond the group of DSM-IV (American Psychiatric Association 1994) anxiety disorders to play a role in many other psychiatric and medical conditions. Pharmacotherapy's roles in ameliorating anxiety, therefore, are often applied to a wide range of diagnoses. The discussion is further broadened because a large variety of medications possess anxiolytic properties. Important treatment roles have emerged for agents specifically designated as *anxiolytics* (to relieve anxiety), others labeled *hypnotics* (sleep inducers), and still others that are in clinical use although they are not specifically labeled for use in the treatment of anxiety.

The decision regarding which medication to use and whether to employ it alone or in combination with other treatments is often complex. Like other clinical decisions, it involves an appraisal of the balance between benefits and risks. Basic but controversial assumptions about the nature of anxiety symptoms also play a role. Whenever possible, clinician and patient should assess the risks and benefits of pharmacotherapy collaboratively.

To support a patient's informed decision regarding treatment, the alternatives, benefits, and risks of pharmacotherapy for anxiety are generally discussed before prescribing. In this discussion, clinician and patient review the usual and/or life-threatening pharmacological adverse effects of specific medications—for example, the small but significant risk of anterograde amnesia with benzodiazepines or of cardiac conduction delays with tricyclic antidepressants (TCAs). Adverse effects vary greatly from drug to drug, and their impact also depends on individual patient characteristics such as age, gender, and concomitant medical illness.

At evaluation for pharmacotherapy, many patients report that they are already taking other prescribed medications or recreational drugs that affect the central nervous system. Another risk of pharmacotherapy, therefore, is the potential interaction of medications with each other or with recreational substances such as alcohol. Some of these interactions can have lethal consequences, such as that of monoamine oxidase inhibitors (MAOIs) with certain foods or prescribed medications. A more common but often less dangerous interaction occurs when certain newer antidepressants (such as fluoxetine or paroxetine) alter the body's metabolism of certain other concurrently used drugs.

An additional concern with pharmacotherapy is the exposure of people to drugs that are potentially abusable, an event that may initiate some new cases of drug abuse. Other patients may not abuse the drugs or become addicted to them in DSM-IV terms, but may nevertheless come to rely upon medication in a psychological sense. This may be an unavoidable consequence of drug efficacy. In assessing the treatment of patients reluctant to discontinue an effective but abusable medication, the controversial distinctions among abuse, addiction, and dependence become very important.

Predisposing risks for developing psychological dependence—a sense of being unable to function without medication—are still poorly understood. Psychotherapists of patients receiving medication often fear that pharmacotherapy will inevitably lead to this type of dependence, altering the patient's capacity to experience life fully or to participate deeply in psychotherapy. Because human growth requires an individual to act in response to anxiety, to experience the consequences of those actions, and to learn from them, patients and therapists alike regard anxiolytic medications with a mixture of appreciation and misgiving.

Even though genetic antecedents of temperament influence an individual's levels of fear and curiosity, the mastery of distressing situations is an important contributor to self-esteem throughout life. The importance of this process is reflected in the effectiveness of *systematic desensitization,* a form of cognitive-behavior therapy (CBT) that offers successively more challenging opportunities for mastery to patients afflicted with anxiety. Some cognitive-behavioral psychotherapists, therefore, have questioned whether the availability of medications that diminish the urgency of psychological problem solving may discourage the attempt to master anxiety through such efforts. Currently available data provide no definitive answer to this question, but my clinical experience has led me to believe that anxiolytic pharmacotherapy does indeed allow some patients to choose symptom relief over a more painful but perhaps more growth-promoting confrontation of psychological issues. Marks (1983) cited uncontrolled evidence that high doses of benzodiazepines may inhibit the effectiveness of exposure treatment for people with phobias. On the other hand, there clearly are some patients for whom nothing but pharmacological intervention will ameliorate symptoms, and some for whom pharmacological intervention is required to even *begin* other interventions. These issues will be discussed later in this chapter.

The benefits of antianxiety pharmacotherapy, like the risks, are multifaceted. An underlying principle, however, is that medications allow many people to overcome anxiety so severe that it had rendered role functioning and even participation in psychotherapy impossible. Controlled clinical studies are still limited, but in one interesting open study (Faigel 1991), 32 students who reported severe examination stress took the Scholastic Aptitude Test (SAT) once, and then again following administration of 40 mg of propranolol 1 hour before the test. Mean SAT scores were increased by 130 points after the propranolol as compared with the first test. These students were not screened for an anxiety diagnosis, but were self-selected as people who felt that their performance on tests was diminished because of anxiety. The range of factors that makes one person's experience of anxiety differ from another's is incompletely understood. The DSM classification of anxiety disorders provides one system for classifying pathological states of anxiety, but misses many nuances appreciated by psychotherapists, who take into account psychodynamic or behavioral factors not included in the DSM's descriptive definitions. As long as treatment involves an individual consideration of each patient's diagnosis, psychodynamics, and history, there will continue to be clinical instances that justify the use of medications to reduce anxiety to a level that permits a fuller participation in life.

An approach I advocate in this chapter is to assess how pharmacotherapy may be integrated with nonsomatic approaches such as exploratory psychotherapy, cognitive therapy, and various behavioral approaches (e.g., relaxation training, biofeedback). Alone or in combination, these treatment modalities may be helpful in alleviating any of the DSM anxiety disorders, anxiety associated with depression or psychosis, or anxiety accompanying a medical disorder. Here I consider generalized anxiety disorder, social phobia, and performance anxiety. I first review each separately as a diagnostic entity, and then examine the available treatments. Finally, I discuss two issues of special concern in pharmacotherapy: the use of anxiolytic medications in pregnant women and the potential for drug dependence.

In integrated treatment, one clinician may provide all modalities or the modalities may be divided among two or more clinicians. In the latter scenario, the fundamental tenet is that integration requires collaboration. Each clinician must appreciate the value of each treatment approach if not all of its technical details. A second tenet of integrative treatment is that the collaboration must also include the patient, who is an active participant in discussions regarding treatment options.

A third tenet of combining therapeutic modalities holds that multiple approaches are clinically justified when the benefit-risk ratio exceeds that associated with the use of a single treatment approach. In practice, choices are often constrained by issues of access, cost, or clinicians' training. The tendency for mental health clinicians to accept a Cartesian split of mind (psychological) versus body (brain), too, may influence treatment choice. A more holistic approach has gained support from recent evidence suggesting that personality is influenced genetically (Lahmeyer et al. 1989; Siever and Davis 1991; Tellegen et al. 1988), that somatic therapies may influence personality (Goldman et al. 1994; Hymowitz et al. 1986), and that nonsomatic therapies may alter brain metabolism in ways similar to somatic therapies (Baxter et al. 1992).

It is useful for clinicians to base their treatment planning on a paradigm that supports their clinical decisions and actions, even if that paradigm turns out to be only partially verifiable. By doing so, clinicians will maintain a framework for communication and for the generation and testing of clinical hypotheses. A caveat regarding paradigms, of course, is that they must be flexible enough to allow reevaluation when clinical response does not occur as expected. The paradigm presented in this chapter endorses the view that distinctions between the psychological and the biochemical are not always clear, so that the common dichotomization of disorders into "biological" and "psychological" must be discarded in favor of a model that recognizes how symptoms and disorders can be simultaneously biological *and* psychological. This broader model, in turn, leads to rejecting the notion that an anxiety disorder represents a "chemical imbalance" that can be expected to respond only to medications, while accepting the idea that medi-

cations can play a useful role even in anxiety disorders that appear
clearly linked to psychosocial stressors. That some disorders may,
in fact, respond better to somatic therapies does not imply that
those disorders involve more of a "chemical imbalance" than others. The ability to appreciate a collaborating therapist's paradigm
is required when multiple caregivers provide different aspects of
treatment. When medication is combined with some form of psychotherapy, it is important for caregivers to discuss among themselves and with their patient whether medication is to be viewed
as a temporary facilitator of psychotherapy or as a longer-term
intervention of greater independence.

A significant advantage of rejecting the Cartesian mind-body
split is that by doing so, one also discards the treatment corollary
of that dichotomization—the assumption that a disorder should be
treated with either psychotherapy or pharmacotherapy but not simultaneously with both modalities. When treatment modalities
are combined, the patient should not be given the impression that
referral of a psychotherapy patient for pharmacotherapy (or the
reverse) represents a clinician's lack of confidence in the initial
treatment approach. In this way, the patient is offered a synergy of
treatments rather than a forced either-or choice. Such an approach
lays the groundwork for true integrative therapy.

Risks and benefits of medications should be discussed as part
of the collaborative treatment planning, and patients should be
involved in evaluating the significance of particular risks and benefits as applied to themselves. A concern commonly voiced by patients who are prescribed antianxiety medications is "If this works,
will I have to be on it forever?" For some patients, combined treatment may act on psychosocial and biochemical functioning in a
way that diminishes the need for further treatment. Others face a
longer-term involvement with one or more therapeutic modalities.
Somatic treatments of anxiety, in general, should be tapered every
6 months to allow clinical reassessment. Ideally, medications can
be tapered slowly and then discontinued for a drug-free interval of
observation; however, some patients' anxiety is so severe that a
taper must be aborted before successful drug discontinuation. If
the taper is sufficiently slow, reemergence of symptoms should be

separable from a drug discontinuation effect. It is often not possible to predict which patients will require the most prolonged treatment.

In summary, integration of modalities can occur when caregivers collaborate with each other, patients are actively involved in decision making, and caregivers espouse a more holistic—as opposed to dualistic—view of mind and brain.

▌ Generalized Anxiety Disorder

The current DSM-IV criteria for generalized anxiety disorder (GAD) (Table 1–1), which evolved from the much earlier concept of "anxiety neurosis," differentiate a condition of chronic free-floating anxiety from the more episodic and intense disturbance of panic disorder. The minimum duration of symptoms required by DSM-IV is 6 months, which is the same interval stipulated in DSM-III-R (American Psychiatric Association 1987) but an increase from the 1 month required by DSM-III (American Psychiatric Association 1980). Another major change in DSM-III-R from DSM-III was the alteration of hierarchical rules so that GAD could be diagnosed in the presence of other Axis I disorders. DSM-IV preserves this convention.

Whereas data have confirmed panic disorder as a discrete illness, GAD has not been proven to be as demonstrably a valid syndrome (DiNardo et al. 1993). Moreover, prevalence data from large-scale population studies have typically used DSM-III criteria, thereby limiting the relevance of these studies to GAD as currently defined. In the discussion that follows, DSM-III criteria are assumed unless other criteria are specified.

A 1979 U.S. survey using a symptom checklist found symptoms comparable to GAD in 6.4% of the adult population (Uhlenhuth et al. 1983). Surprisingly, this study noted that only 27% of persons diagnosable with GAD were taking antianxiety medication. In the Epidemiologic Catchment Area (ECA) program of the National Institute of Mental Heath the 1-year prevalence for GAD

Table 1–1.   DSM-IV diagnostic criteria for generalized anxiety
                  disorder

A. Excessive anxiety and worry (apprehensive expectation), occurring
    more days than not for at least 6 months, about a number of
    events or activities (such as work or school performance).

B. The person finds it difficult to control the worry.

C. The anxiety and worry are associated with three (or more) of the
    following six symptoms (with at least some symptoms present for
    more days than not for the past 6 months).   **Note:** Only one
    item is required in children.

    (1)   restlessness or feeling keyed up or on edge

    (2)   being easily fatigued

    (3)   difficulty concentrating or mind going blank

    (4)   irritability

    (5)   muscle tension

    (6)   sleep disturbance (difficulty falling or staying asleep, or
          restless unsatisfying sleep)

D. The focus of the anxiety and worry is not confined to features of
    an Axis I disorder, e.g., the anxiety or worry is not about having a
    panic attack (as in panic disorder), being embarrassed in public (as
    in social phobia), being contaminated (as in obsessive-compulsive
    disorder), being away from home or close relatives (as in separation
    anxiety disorder), gaining weight (as in anorexia nervosa), having
    multiple physical complaints (as in somatization disorder), or
    having a serious illness (as in hypochondriasis), and the anxiety
    and worry do not occur exclusively during posttraumatic stress
    disorder.

E. The anxiety, worry, or physical symptoms cause clinically
    significant distress or impairment in social, occupational, or other
    important areas of functioning.

F. The disturbance is not due to the direct physiological effects of a
    substance (e.g., a drug of abuse, a medication) or a general medical
    condition (e.g., hyperthyroidism) and does not occur exclusively
    during a mood disorder, a psychotic disorder, or a pervasive
    developmental disorder.

Source.   Reprinted from American Psychiatric Association: *Diagnostic
and Statistical Manual of Mental Disorders, 4th Edition.* Washington, DC,
American Psychiatric Association, 1994, pp. 435–436. Used with
permission.

in the population subset from the St. Louis, Missouri, area was estimated to be 1.8% in men, 2.6% in women, and 2.3% overall (Blazer et al. 1987). The most recent figures come from the National Comorbidity Survey (NCS; Wittchen et al. 1994), and show a current prevalence for DSM-III-R GAD of 1.6% of people aged 15–54 years in this large, population-based survey. Twelve-month prevalence was 3.1% and lifetime prevalence was 5.1%.

Blazer and colleagues (1987) demonstrated a correlation between the risk for GAD and the number of recent stressful life events. In men, the presence of four or more such events was associated with a risk for GAD 8.5 times that for men with three or fewer events. In women, however, no such association was found. These data raise the intriguing hypothesis that GAD differs between men and women.

A recent family study of GAD in women assessed heritability of the disorder using DSM-III-R criteria. By studying 1,033 female–female twin pairs, an estimate was made that the heritability of GAD may be as high as 30%. This study's results also suggested that in this group of women, liability to major depression and to GAD were influenced by the same genetic factors (Kendler et al. 1992a).

The etiology of GAD is complex and appears to involve at least the gamma-aminobutyric acid (GABA), noradrenergic, and serotonergic neurotransmitter systems (Nutt 1990). A topographic electroencephalogram (EEG) study comparing 19 GAD subjects with 11 control subjects noted differences in the EEG response to light, a finding interpreted as evidence of a decreased level of attention to external stimuli resulting from competition with internal processes (Grillon and Buchsbaum 1987). Studies using a rodent model of anxiety have associated social stress in mice with increased cortical levels of messenger RNA (mRNA) for $alpha_1$ and $gamma_2$ subunits of the $GABA_A$ receptor complex (Miller and Kastin 1991). It is worth restating that physiological markers of GAD may reflect genetic vulnerabilities, responses to environmental factors, or both.

Comorbidity of GAD with other psychiatric disorders is high. In one study, among patients who had experienced GAD sometime in their lifetime, the level of comorbidity with other psychiatric illnesses was 90.4% (Wittchen et al. 1994). In an earlier study, 42% of 109 subjects with GAD had experienced at least one major depressive episode during their lifetime. Twenty-three percent had concurrent social phobia, and 21% had concurrent simple phobia (Brawman et al. 1993). Of 79 GAD patients given a dexamethasone suppression test, 27% were nonsuppressors, a rate the authors found comparable to that for outpatients with depression and higher than that for panic disorder patients (Miller et al. 1986).

GAD has also been associated with Axis II disorders. In a subpopulation (Eastern Baltimore, Maryland) of the ECA study, the relationship between personality disorders and DSM-III Axis I diagnoses was examined (Nestadt et al. 1992). High scores for compulsive personality were significantly correlated with diagnoses of GAD or simple phobia but with smaller odds of having alcohol use disorders. In contrast, high antisocial personality scores predicted alcohol use disorders but a lower risk for GAD.

Research into the pharmacotherapy of GAD has extensively addressed the effects of benzodiazepines, buspirone, and antidepressants. Other medications that have received attention include neuroleptics and several drugs now in clinical trials (e.g., gepirone, an azapirone similar to buspirone). The widespread applicability of drug research findings has been questioned because of the tendency for researchers to examine samples of individuals who, having been recruited through advertisements, may differ greatly from those seen in naturalistic treatment settings. Although such recruitment is performed to facilitate the research process, it is my experience that patients seeking or already receiving treatment outside of a research protocol tend to have several disorders rather than a single diagnostic entity and to suffer greater disability than recruited subjects. In community surveys, too, comorbidity is higher than would be predicted by chance (Caron and Rutter 1991). Having stated these limitations, I will nonetheless review the pharmacotherapeutic treatment options suggested by research on GAD.

At present, the benzodiazepines (BZDs) have the widest clinical use in GAD treatment. These agents are effective and relatively safe, and exert prolonged antianxiety effects. Though equally powerful in counteracting anxiety symptoms, the various BZDs differ in potency, half-life, and metabolism in ways that affect treatment planning. The frequency of adverse effects, too, may differ from one BZD to another. One adverse effect of particular concern with patients receiving concurrent psychotherapy is anterograde amnesia, because its occurrence could theoretically impair a patient's capacity to benefit from a psychotherapy session. Anterograde amnesia is most profound with the shorter-acting drugs of this class (Kanno et al. 1993; Mejo 1992; Shader and Greenblatt 1983).

Buspirone, an azapirone, requires 1–3 weeks to achieve its clinical effects, a period similar to that required by the TCAs. After this latency period, buspirone is as effective as diazepam in ameliorating GAD symptoms (Feighner et al. 1982; Rickels et al. 1988). No objective data support the notion that buspirone would be a better medication than a benzodiazepine to combine with CBT, but many clinicians have welcomed buspirone's apparent lack of abuse potential.

TCAs are frequently used in treating anxiety symptoms. Although these agents possess specific antipanic effects, their effects on the symptoms of GAD are more diffuse. It is possible that sedative effects play an important role, or that the effects of antidepressants on GAD indicate a pathophysiological relationship between GAD and depression. In a 6-week double-blind parallel-design study with flexible dosage scheduling (Hoehn-Saric et al. 1988), imipramine was compared with alprazolam in 60 patients with GAD. The authors found that the two drugs resulted in comparable improvement after 2 weeks as measured by rating scales that assessed both psychic and somatic symptoms. Alprazolam was more effective in relieving somatic symptoms, whereas imipramine was more effective in relieving psychic symptoms such as dysphoria or negative anticipatory thinking. Antidepressants may be especially effective in patients who show a mixed anxious-depressed state. Cardiac and other adverse effects make these drugs more problematic than the BZDs from a medical perspective, but as with buspirone, there is little potential for abuse.

Antihistamines exert a sedating effect that is much less specific than that of the BZDs in alleviating anxiety. The principal advantage of these agents is their low liability for abuse. Because antihistamines produce sedative effects, there is reason to wonder about their potential for interference in CBT or other treatment processes that require attentiveness. Unlike the BZDs, they have not been shown to induce amnestic states.

Neuroleptics, which are primarily used in the treatment of psychosis, have significant short- and long-term toxicity. In low doses, they can relieve anxiety (Heinrich and Lehman 1991; Proctor 1960). One neuroleptic, trifluoperazine, has been shown to be effective in treating GAD (Heinrich and Lehman 1991; Mendels et al. 1986); it is the only neuroleptic approved by the U.S. Food and Drug Administration (FDA) for treatment of anxiety. The short- and long-term toxic effects of neuroleptics limit their clinical usefulness.

Studies that have compared psychotherapy with pharmacotherapy have found the two modalities to be equally effective in the treatment of GAD (Lindsay et al. 1987; Tyrer et al. 1988). A recent literature review of psychological treatments of GAD concluded that such treatments can result in mean reductions of 50% in the severity of somatic symptoms, a 25% reduction in a measure of trait anxiety, and achievement of "normal functioning" in approximately 50% of patients (Durham and Allan 1993). The authors also noted that better psychotherapy outcomes occurred in studies that recruited subjects from primary care settings who were medication-free when they entered the study. It is not clear whether these findings were biased by referral of patients who differ from those usually seen by mental health clinicians. In a mental health setting, symptoms may be severe enough to require combinations of pharmacotherapy and psychotherapy, and this combined treatment may even be needed indefinitely by some patients (Rickels and Schweizer 1990).

Another potentially confounding variable is what is meant by the term *psychotherapy* as reported in various studies. Sometimes it was specified as CBT, insight-oriented therapy, interpersonal therapy, or any of a variety of time-limited therapies. British reports tend to assume CBT, and as a whole, the nature of clinical research favors the use of short-term treatments as the "psychotherapy component" in this sort of trial. The reasons for this preference include the short-term funding of research and the greater ease of standardizing CBT techniques.

▌ Social Phobia

Social phobia (SP) has been less frequently diagnosed than GAD, but the most recent community study estimated its lifetime prevalence to be 13.3% (Rapaport 1994; Wittchen et al. 1994), a figure more than four times as high as previous estimates (Agras 1990; Pollard and Henderson 1990; Regier et al. 1988). This higher rate has been explained by the inclusion of younger respondents in the newer study. Given the early age at onset associated with SP, such a difference would have a considerable impact. ECA data from 13,000 adults in four U.S. communities showed higher rates of SP among women, younger adults (ages 18–29 years), the less educated, and people of lower socioeconomic status. Mean age at onset was 15.5 years, and onset later than 25 years of age was uncommon. In contrast to persons with no psychiatric disorders, those with SP showed increased rates of suicidal ideation, financial dependency, and utilization of medical services, but not higher rates of suicide attempts or of help seeking from mental health professionals (Schneier et al. 1992). Another ECA report, perhaps as a result of study population differences, could not confirm the higher rate of SP among women (Bourdon et al. 1988).

DSM-IV distinguishes two types of SP on the basis of whether anxiety-provoking situations are generalized or differentiated (as in public speaking) (see Table 1–2). Although this distinction has been disputed, at least one study has demonstrated differences between these two proposed subtypes. In one study, 35 subjects with the generalized subtype of SP were compared with 22 others with the differentiated type (in this case, anxiety related to public speaking). The generalized subjects were younger, less educated, and ✻

Table 1–2. DSM-IV diagnostic criteria for social phobia

A. A marked and persistent fear of one or more social or performance situations in which the person is exposed to unfamiliar people or to possible scrutiny by others. The individual fears that he or she will act in a way (or show anxiety symptoms) that will be humiliating or embarrassing. **Note:** In children, there must be evidence of the capacity for age-appropriate social relationships with familiar people and the anxiety must occur in peer settings, not just in interactions with adults.

B. Exposure to the feared social situation almost invariably provokes anxiety, which may take the form of a situationally bound or situationally predisposed panic attack. **Note:** In children, the anxiety may be expressed by crying, tantrums, freezing, or shrinking from social situations with unfamiliar people.

C. The person recognizes that the fear is excessive or unreasonable. **Note:** In children, this feature may be absent.

D. The feared social or performance situations are avoided or else are endured with intense anxiety or distress.

E. The avoidance, anxious anticipation, or distress in the feared social or performance situation(s) interferes significantly with the person's normal routine, occupational (academic) functioning, or social activities or relationships, or there is marked distress about having the phobia.

F. In individuals under age 18 years, the duration is at least 6 months.

G. The fear or avoidance is not due to the direct physiological effects of a substance (e.g., a drug of abuse, a medication) or a general medical condition and is not better accounted for by another mental disorder (e.g., panic disorder with or without agoraphobia, separation anxiety disorder, body dysmorphic disorder, a pervasive developmental disorder, or schizoid personality disorder).

H. If a general medical condition or another mental disorder is present, the fear in criterion A is unrelated to it, e.g., the fear is not of stuttering, trembling in Parkinson's disease, or exhibiting abnormal eating behavior in anorexia nervosa or bulimia nervosa.

Specify if:

Generalized: if the fears include most social situations (also consider the additional diagnosis of avoidant personality disorder)

Source. Reprinted from American Psychiatric Association: *Diagnostic and Statistical Manual of Mental Disorders, 4th Edition.* Washington, DC, American Psychiatric Association, 1994, pp. 416–417. Used with permission.

less likely to be employed than the differentiated ones (Heimberg et al. 1990). A retrospective comparison of subjects with generalized SP and with differentiated SP found the number of subjects with a history of depression to be comparable, with 37% for the former and 30% for the latter (Stein et al. 1990). Although the differentiated type of anxiety can resemble the syndrome of "performance anxiety," it is typically associated with far more disability. It is likely that many people who consider themselves to have performance anxiety meet the DSM-III-R criteria for SP (Clark and Agras 1991).

A number of studies have attempted to elucidate SP's heritability. In one study (Fyer et al. 1993), first-degree relatives of persons with SP meeting the DSM-III-R criteria were compared with first-degree relatives of persons who had received a diagnosis of a mental illness. Relatives of persons with SP were more likely to have received a diagnosis of SP (16% versus 5%; relative risk = 3.12) but were no more likely to have received a diagnosis of another anxiety disorder than were relatives of non-SP individuals. An earlier family-history study (Reich and Yates 1988a) showed a suggestive, though not statistically significant, similar trend. In a study of 2,163 female twins (Kendler et al. 1992a), the authors estimated the liability for genetic heritability of agoraphobia, simple phobia, and social phobia to range from 30% to 40%. Using multivariate genetic modeling, the authors suggested that environmental experiences that predispose to all phobias were most relevant for SP and agoraphobia. Approaching this issue from another direction, investigators (Biederman et al. 1990; Kagan et al. 1988; Rosenbaum et al. 1991) have demonstrated an increased risk for anxiety disorders, including SP, among children with the stable, observable trait of *behavioral inhibition*. Taken together, these findings suggest that SP is a disorder distinct from other anxiety disorders, and that a genetically transmitted vulnerability is involved.

The search for physiological markers of SP has produced both positive and negative findings. No differences in plasma T3, T4, free T4, or thyroid-stimulating hormone (TSH) levels were found when patients with SP were compared with age- and sex-matched control subjects (Tancer et al. 1990). Since cortisol is produced in response to stress, urinary free cortisol was measured in 10 patients with SP and 15 age- and sex-matched control subjects (Potts et al. 1991). No differences in cortisol or in the ratio of free cortisol to creatinine were found. Lactate infusion, which often induces a panic attack in panic disorder patients, resulted in a panic attack in only 1 of 15 patients with SP (Liebowitz et al. 1985). The hypothesized association between SP and altered adrenergic function was examined in an open study of 11 patients meeting the DSM-III-R criteria for SP. In this study, only one SP patient experienced observable anxiety in response to an epinephrine infusion (Papp et al. 1988).

The search for biological markers, however, has identified a few promising leads. For example, some people with SP show a blunted biochemical response to challenge with clonidine, an alpha$_2$-adrenergic agonist (Uhde et al. 1991). Another suggestive finding is the measurement of significantly higher plasma norepinephrine levels in response to postural blood pressure changes in 14 subjects with SP compared with 14 matched control subjects and 14 other matched subjects with panic disorder (Stein et al. 1992).

Early attempts to explain the pathophysiology of SP proposed that the subjective experience of anxiety resulted when an individual became aware of the physiological changes associated with adrenergic hyperactivity, such as dry mouth, palpitations, and tremor (see Chapter 8). The logical deduction was to treat SP with drugs that blocked beta-adrenergic receptors. These drugs have been shown to be more effective than placebo but less effective than phenelzine, an MAOI (Liebowitz et al. 1986, 1991). Somatic anxiety responds more fully than does subjective (psychic) anxiety to beta-blockers (Brantigan et al. 1979, 1982). One recent controlled study (Liebowitz et al. 1991) confirmed that SP can respond to treatment with atenolol, but—at least in this group of patients—the effect was less robust than that achieved with phenelzine. In this study, the response rates measured were 23% for placebo, 30% for atenolol, and 64% for phenelzine. Phenelzine has also been compared with cognitive-behavioral group therapy, alprazolam, and pill-placebo plus instructions for self-directed exposure in patients with SP (Gelernter et al. 1991). All approaches produced significant improvement, with only minor differences. An open study (Heimberg et al. 1985) examining treatment of SP with exposure, cognitive restructuring, and homework assignments found that significant gains were made by most patients and were maintained at 3- and 6-month follow-ups.

Preliminary evidence suggests that fluoxetine, a selective serotonin reuptake inhibitor (SSRI), is effective in treating SP (Black and Tancer 1992; Wittchen and Essau 1993). Fluoxetine was administered to 16 patients with DSM-III-R–defined SP in a 12-week open clinical trial. Of the 13 patients who remained throughout the trial (3 dropped out because of adverse effects), 10 were considered to be responders and 3, nonresponders (Wittchen and Essau 1993). Sertraline, another SSRI, has shown efficacy in preliminary open trials (Czepowicz et al. 1994; Martins et al. 1994). The effects of paroxetine, venlafaxine, fluvoxamine, and nefazodone remain to be investigated.

In an open pilot study with alprazolam, various measures of symptoms and disability improved but returned to baseline after the drug was withdrawn (Reich and Yates 1988b). In another study, alprazolam was used to treat 14 people with SP by DSM-III-R criteria. Six of nine avoidant personality traits improved with treatment, but all but one (avoiding social or occupational activities requiring interpersonal contact) returned to baseline following discontinuation (Reich et al. 1989).

Clonazepam was used to treat 26 outpatients with SP in an open naturalistic study (Davidson et al. 1991). At follow-up evaluation (after an average of 11.3 months of treatment), 84.6% showed "good improvement," and 14.4% "showed no improvement or were not recovered." The mean dose declined over time from a peak of 2.1 mg/day to 0.94 mg/day. In another naturalistic study (Reiter et al. 1990), 9 out of 11 patients with SP responded to treatment with clonazepam at 0.75–3.00 mg/day. In a third open study (Munjack et al. 1990), 23 patients with SP were randomly assigned to 8 weeks of clonazepam or a nontreatment control group. The clonazepam group experienced significant improvement on a variety of measures.

In summary, there is good evidence for the efficacies of phenelzine, clonazepam, and/or CBT in the treatment of SP, and preliminary evidence suggests that fluoxetine and sertraline are effective as well. Longer-term follow-up studies are needed, however, to clarify whether these treatments produce changes that are maintained beyond the period of treatment. Only one open study (Heimberg et al. 1985) has approached this question for CBT, and although promising results were obtained, follow-up with controlled studies is needed. Alprazolam is effective, but it is also unclear how long benefits can be expected to persist beyond the treatment period.

▌ Performance Anxiety

Performance anxiety is a syndrome, typically described by performers, consisting of subjective anxiety associated with physical symptoms such as palpitations, dry mouth, sweating, and tremor. In a survey of the International Group of Performing Artists, 27% of the respondents reported occasional uses of a beta-blocker for performance anxiety (Fishbein et al. 1988). Beta-blockers are useful in moderating heart rate and decreasing dry mouth and tremor. They are less useful in relieving subjective anxiety (Brantigan et al. 1979, 1982). Performance anxiety in 33 young string-playing music students was treated with 40 mg of nadolol (a beta-blocker) or 2 mg of diazepam in a double-blind, crossover study (James and Savage 1984). Subjective experience of anxiety was unchanged in both groups, but nadolol attenuated the rise in pulse associated with anxiety and improved aspects of playing that were felt to be adversely affected by tremor. Diazepam caused a minor deterioration in performance.

In another study using nadolol, 34 singing students were given either placebo or nadolol (20, 40, or 80 mg) in a double-blind crossover design (Gates et al. 1985). Low-dose nadolol enhanced performance, whereas higher doses impaired performance.

Buspirone was compared with a 5-session, group CBT program in a double-blind crossover study of 94 subjects with performance anxiety (Clark and Agras 1991). Subjects were recruited through mass-media announcements and met the DSM-III-R criteria for SP. CBT but not buspirone resulted in improved performance confidence and improved quality of musical performance.

In contrast to their more modest effects on SP, beta-blockers appear highly effective in the treatment of performance anxiety, although there appears to be a limit beyond which dosage increases may cause decrements in performance. CBT, too, appears efficacious.

▌ Overview of Anxiolytic Medication Properties

Medications differ in mechanism of action, specific efficacy, adverse effects, and other attributes. Placing the properties of available medications into a broader conceptual framework proves useful when considering their use in combination with other therapies. One major distinction to be made is between drugs that exert their effects for a brief time after ingestion of a single dose, such as benzodiazepines and beta-blockers, and those that generally require daily ingestion over days to weeks in order to exert their effects, such as antidepressants or buspirone. In the first group, patients more readily perceive the relationship between taking the drug and feeling the clinical effects. The patient's experience is that the effect is contingent on ingesting the drug, and so, for ease of discussion, this group of medications will be referred to as contingent-effect (CE) drugs. Patients experience an effect from the second group after a latency period, and thus these medications will be referred to as latent-effect (LE) drugs.

CE drugs are sometimes prescribed on an "as needed" basis. Although patients taking these drugs may regard their effects as positive, some psychotherapists worry that CE drugs can introduce an obstacle into the psychotherapy process. Patients who are prescribed CE drugs may have more difficulty with psychotherapies that require exposure or the learning of new cognitive skills if they can choose to bypass the effort of employing a new thought or action pattern by simply taking the medicine. One way to circumvent this potential problem is to prescribe CE medicines on a fixed schedule so that flexibility of dosing is eliminated. In my clinical experience, such a strategy can be useful, but its efficacy awaits confirmation from controlled clinical trials. The LE drugs present far less of this particular problem and for this reason are generally more easily combined with psychotherapeutic approaches.

A second distinction can be made between drugs with and without significant abuse potential. With some exceptions, LE drugs have less potential for dependency or abuse than do CE drugs. One exception to this generalization is the class of beta-blockers, which is in the CE group but not typically abused. On the other hand, tranylcypromine, in the LE group, is an occasionally abused drug (Briggs et al. 1990).

Antidepressants

Tricyclic Antidepressants

TCAs are efficacious in the treatment of panic disorder, anxiety with depression, and GAD. In the treatment of panic disorder, cumulative clinical experience with these drugs exceeds that with all other drugs combined. Another tricyclic, clomipramine, is useful in the treatment of obsessive-compulsive disorder. Some of these drugs are quite sedating, a property that can be helpful when insomnia is a symptom.

The TCAs were introduced in the 1950s, beginning with imipramine, a drug structurally similar to chlorpromazine. The eight TCAs available in the United States today can be subdivided into two groups based on a structural distinction having to do with how many methyl groups are bound to a terminal nitrogen (Table 1–3). The classification into *tertiary* or *secondary* amines is useful in predicting clinical properties and adverse effects. Amitriptyline, imipramine, clomipramine, and doxepin are tertiary amines, whereas desipramine, nortriptyline, protriptyline, and amoxapine are secondary amines.

All TCAs block the synaptic reuptake of certain neurotransmitters. The tertiary amines are more selective for serotonin (5-hydroxytryptamine, or 5-HT) as compared with the secondary amines. This property and differences in lipid solubility may account for the tertiary amines' more prominent adverse effects. All TCAs are metabolized by hepatic microsomal systems, and the tertiary amines are metabolized first into compounds that are themselves clinically active. Thus, imipramine is metabolized to desipramine, and amitriptyline to nortriptyline. Absorption from the gastrointestinal tract is usually complete, but differences in hepatic metabolism and protein binding result in significant variations in serum levels among individuals given the same dose. Serum levels can be commercially obtained for most of the TCAs and are often useful in determining dosage. With the exception of nortriptyline, which has an inverted U-shaped dose-response curve, dose-response curves are sigmoid-shaped. This means that despite variations in metabolism and serum binding, doses can often be adjusted appropriately on the basis of clinical observation alone. With nortriptyline, however, because of its different dose-response curve, serum levels may be useful in determining the optimal dose.

Adverse effects of the TCAs include orthostatic hypotension, sedation, cardiac conduction delay, and anticholinergic effects such as dry mouth, constipation, blurred vision, and urinary retention. Anticholinergic effects, sedation, and orthostatic hypotension are greater with the tertiary amines than with the secondary amines. These adverse effects can be minimized by starting at low doses and titrating carefully upward with appropriate monitoring.

Another adverse effect is related to TCAs' mechanism of therapeutic action. Reuptake blockade initially results in more neurotransmitter being present at the synapse, which is followed by downregulation of presynaptic and postsynaptic receptors and normalization of neurotransmitter levels. This downregulation is chronologically related to clinical response. In the time that pre-

Table 1–3. Tricyclic antidepressants (TCAs) (selective listing)

Type	Generic name	Trade name	Dose range (mg/day)	Effective plasma level (ng/ml)
Tertiary amines	Amitriptyline	Elavil	50–300	> 120
	Imipramine	Tofranil	50–300	> 225
	Clomipramine	Anafranil	50–250	
	Doxepin	Sinequan, Adapin	25–300	100–250
	Trimipramine	Surmontil	50–300	
Secondary amines	Nortriptyline	Pamelor, Aventyl	25–150	50–150
	Desipramine	Norpramin, Pertofrane	50–300	> 125

Note. Many of these agents are available generically.

cedes normalization of neurotransmitter levels, patients may experience adverse effects of increased anxiety, tremor, and restlessness—a symptom cluster that has been termed the *early tricyclic syndrome* (Pollack and Rosenbaum 1987; Rosenbaum 1984) and that is most prominent with the secondary amines. Because this cluster of potential adverse effects can be particularly disturbing for patients with anxiety disorders, TCAs should be started in smaller doses and titrated upward more slowly.

Selective Serotonin Reuptake Inhibitors

In contrast to the effects of TCAs on a variety of neurotransmitters, those of the SSRIs involve more (but not completely) selective blocking of the reuptake of 5-HT. The four SSRIs currently available on the U.S. market are fluoxetine (Prozac), sertraline (Zoloft), paroxetine (Paxil), and fluvoxamine (Luvox). Another drug that recently became available is venlafaxine (Effexor), which is harder to classify because although it is a potent serotonin reuptake inhibitor and has an adverse effect profile similar to that of the SSRIs, it also blocks norepinephrine and dopamine reuptake. Nefazodone (marketed as Serzone) is a serotonin reuptake blocking antidepressant that also possesses some postsynaptic serotonin antagonist properties, a characteristic that may alter its side-effect profile. (Table 1–4 lists SSRIs currently available in the United States.) The SSRIs differ in structure from the TCAs and also from each other. All of them are effective antidepressants, several of them are also effective in treating panic disorder (Chapter 2) and obsessive-compulsive disorder (Chapter 6), and preliminary evidence suggests that sertraline is effective in treating SP. Other uses of SSRI antidepressants appear promising and await further investigation.

The SSRIs lack the cardiac toxicity of the TCAs, and most also lack anticholinergic adverse effects. Although they are generally well tolerated, adverse effects common to this group include nausea, headache, insomnia, dry mouth, and restlessness, especially at the beginning of treatment. The SSRIs are all LE drugs and may therefore be less likely to interfere with CBT. In fact, the latency

Table 1–4. Selective serotonin reuptake inhibitors (SSRIs) (selective listing)

Generic name	Trade name	Dose range (mg/day)	Half-life (hours)	Half-life of active metabolite
Fluoxetine	Prozac	5–100	48–96	7–15 days
Sertraline	Zoloft	25–200	24	2–4 days
Paroxetine	Paxil	10–50	24	None
Venlafaxine	Effexor	75–225	3–5	9–11 hours
Fluvoxamine	Luvox	100–300	15	None
Nefazodone	Serzone	100–600	2–4	18–33 hours

for efficacy in fluoxetine can be as much as 6–12 weeks, although 4–6 weeks is more common. For the other SSRIs, a shorter period appears to apply. An average daily dose is 20 mg for either fluoxetine or paroxetine, and approximately 50–150 mg for sertraline. Venlafaxine is prescribed in doses from 37.5 to 375 mg/day, and fluvoxamine typically from 100 to 300 mg/day. Nefazodone doses may range from 50 mg bid to as high as 300 mg bid. Initial restlessness can be managed with a benzodiazepine or beta-blocker and usually subsides within a week of treatment. As with the TCAs, adverse effects can be minimized by starting at low doses and titrating gradually upward. Fluoxetine and paroxetine strongly inhibit the IID6 isozyme of the hepatic P-450 cytochrome system; as a consequence, hepatic biotransformation and elimination of drugs metabolized by this isozyme would be expected to decrease, with resultant higher serum levels for any given dose (Crewe et al. 1992). Drugs so affected include some antidepressants (e.g., TCAs), the phenothiazines, and the type 1C antiarrhythmics (propafenone, flecainide, and encainide).

Monoamine Oxidase Inhibitors

The MAOIs are effective in the treatment of panic disorder, mixed depression-anxiety states (Quitkin et al. 1979; Sheehan et al. 1980), and SP (Liebowitz et al. 1992). They may also be effective in certain patients with obsessive-compulsive disorder accompanied by phobic anxiety and/or panic attacks (Jenike et al. 1983) and in bulimia (Stewart et al. 1984), although these uses have not been as rigorously explored. The MAOIs are effective antidepressants (Quitkin et al. 1979) and may be particularly helpful in treating atypical depression (Nies 1984). Because of clinical perceptions about their adverse effects and interactions with other drugs, these agents are rarely used as the first-choice therapy for depressive or anxiety disorders (Clary et al. 1990; Paykel and White 1991) even though they may be effective where other drugs fail.

Monoamine oxidase (MAO) is a mitochondria-linked enzyme distributed widely throughout the body. It oxidizes certain molecules that possess a single amine group, including norepinephrine, dopamine, 5-HT, and tyramine. There are at least two varieties, or *isozymes,* of MAO that differ in distribution and preferred substrates. These are designated MAO-A and MAO-B (Tipton et al. 1983).

The recent withdrawal of isocarboxazid (Marplan) has left three MAOIs available on the U.S. market (Table 1–5). Phenelzine (Nardil) and tranylcypromine (Parnate) affect both MAO-A and MAO-B and are therefore called nonselective MAO inhibitors. Phenelzine, which is structurally related to a hepatotoxic chemical, hydrazine, is potentially more dangerous to the liver than tranylcypromine. A more recently introduced MAOI, selegiline (Deprenyl), has been adopted into psychopharmacological use in the attempt to obtain the behavioral effects of an MAOI while avoiding the risk of a hypertensive crisis. MAO-A, which has a significant representation in the gut wall and liver, oxidizes tyramine, an indirect sympathomimetic amine capable of interacting with nonselective MAOIs to produce a hypertensive crisis. Selegiline at low doses leaves intestinal MAO-A relatively intact, affecting predominantly MAO-B. Although it was approved by the FDA for the treatment of Parkinson's disease, selegiline is also known to produce psychotropic effects at serum levels below those associated with hypertensive reactions in response to tyramine (Mann et al. 1989). Unfortunately, at some higher doses often needed for psychotropic (as compared with antiparkinsonian) effects, it too, inhibits intestinal MAO-A.

Phenelzine and tranylcypromine are irreversible MAOIs. Phenelzine is a longer-acting drug than tranylcypromine. A new generation of reversible and therefore shorter-acting MAOIs, selective for MAO-A, is being developed. Moclobemide, the best known of these, is not currently available for clinical use in the United States. This reversible inhibitor of MAO-A (RIMA) has shown much less propensity for precipitating hypertensive crises (Da Prada et al. 1990) or for causing adverse interactions with other drugs (Dingemanse 1993). The reason for moclobemide's reduced potential for hypertensive effects is not its selectivity but rather its short duration of action.

The chief advantage of the MAOIs is their proven efficacy, especially in the treatment of panic disorder. They also have low abuse potential, although there have been some cases reported of tranylcypromine abuse (Briggs et al. 1990). In addition, they are relatively unlikely to interfere with other treatment modalities. Their disadvantages include a broad range of adverse effects such as hypotension, anorgasmia, impotence, weight gain, hypomania, seizures, urinary retention, and paresthesias (Rabkin et al. 1984). Other serious problems include interactions with foods or beverages containing tyramine or with a number of over-the-counter or prescribed medications, including the sympathomimetic amines—for example, stimulants or phenylpropanolamine; many other antidepressants; the cough suppressant dextromethorphan; and the analgesic meperidine. These interactions can result in symptoms that range from mild headache to more serious, poten-

Table 1–5. Monoamine oxidase inhibitors (MAOIs) (selective listing)

Type	Generic name	Trade name	Dose range (mg/day)
Nonreversible inhibition			
Nonselective	Phenelzine	Nardil	15–90 (approx. 1 mg/kg)
	Tranylcypromine	Parnate	30–60
Selective			
MAO-B selective	Selegiline	Eldepryl, Deprenyl	10–40
Reversible inhibition			
Selective			
MAO-A selective (RIMA)	Moclobemide	*	150–800

Note. RIMA = reversible inhibitor of MAO-A. *Moclobemide is not currently marketed in the United States, although it is marketed in other countries.

tially life-threatening elevations of blood pressure.

The most common adverse effect of MAOIs is postural hypotension. The frequency of this adverse effect can be mitigated by slowly increasing titration of the dosage. Dosage is best established for phenelzine at approximately 1 mg/kg of lean body weight. Patients should be instructed about dietary restrictions and drug interactions. The diet should start at least 3 days before initiation of treatment and continue for 2 weeks following cessation of treatment.

Atypical Antidepressants

This residual group contains only one member used in the treatment of anxiety disorders: trazodone (Desyrel). Like the TCAs, trazodone affects multiple neurotransmitter systems. It is more selective for 5-HT than the TCAs and less so than the SSRIs. It is also fairly sedating, and thus may be used as a hypnotic. Antidepressant doses range from 300 to 600 mg/day, but doses required for sleep-inducing effects are smaller, between 25 mg and 200 mg at bedtime. Trazodone has also proven to be particularly useful in treating the insomnia that is often an adverse effect of fluoxetine. As with antihistamines, it is nonspecifically sedating rather than truly anxiolytic, although it has been used for daytime anxiolysis in alcohol-dependent patients.

Antihistamines

The main therapeutic action of the antihistamines is to block the effects of the neurotransmitter histamine at its postsynaptic receptors. There are at least two classes of histamine receptors: the H_2 receptors mediate gastric acid secretion, and the H_1 receptors are involved in the immune system. Drugs that block the former (e.g., cimetidine, ranitidine) are usually called H_2 blockers, and drugs that block the latter are usually referred to generically as antihistamines. The adverse effects of antihistamines include sedation, dizziness, and postural hypotension. The antihistamines' sedating qualities make them very suitable for use as hypnotics. Their chief value is their low abuse potential, although they are CE drugs. In patients being treated for inflammatory conditions (e.g., allergic rhinitis), sedation can be a troublesome adverse effect. Newer antihistamines that do not penetrate the central nervous system as readily, and that are therefore less sedating, are consequently more useful as antiinflammatory agents than as antianxiety drugs. Table 1–6 lists antihistamines currently available in the United States.

Azapirones

This class currently contains one available member, buspirone (BuSpar), but another azapirone, gepirone, has already reached an advanced stage of clinical testing. Buspirone is a partial agonist at 5-HT$_{1A}$ receptors and appears to work by altering serotonergic neurotransmission. It is well absorbed through the gastrointestinal tract. Its metabolism and elimination involve both the liver and the kidneys. Studies have suggested no potential for abuse, and adverse effects are minimal—headache, nausea, and dizziness. Buspirone's efficacy in treating generalized anxiety has been demonstrated in open and double-blind studies (Feighner 1987; Feighner et al. 1982; Gammans et al. 1992; Rickels and Schweizer 1993). Like that of the antidepressants, its efficacy requires several weeks of treatment and anxiolysis does not rapidly follow individual doses. Most patients can be started on 5 mg bid, and this dosage can be increased as high as 10 mg qid. The maximum recommended dose is 60 mg/day, although recent evidence suggests that there may be antidepressant effects at even higher dosages. Clinicians should be aware that there is no cross-tolerance

Table 1–6. Antihistamines (selective listing)

Generic name	Trade name	Dose range
Hydroxyzine HCl	Atarax	50–100 mg qid
Hydroxyzine pamoate	Vistaril	50–100 mg qid
Diphenhydramine	Benadryl	25–50 mg qid

Note. These agents are also available generically.

between buspirone and BZDs, so buspirone cannot be used to treat BZD withdrawal (Schweizer and Rickels 1986).

Buspirone's major advantages are its lack of abuse potential and the fact that it is an LE drug. It also has less-frequent adverse effects on memory than do the BZDs (Galpern et al. 1988; Wu et al. 1987). The major disadvantages of buspirone are that its long latency for effect makes it useless for acute anxiolysis and that patients who have previously been treated with BZDs tend to prefer BZD effects over those of buspirone (Biederman and Jellinek 1986).

Imidazopyradines

At present, only one imidazopyridine (zolpidem) is marketed in the United States, and the FDA indication for its use is as a sleep-inducing agent (hypnotic). Marketed under the trade name of Ambien, zolpidem is not a BZD but rather is a specific agonist of omega$_1$ benzodiazepine receptors (Roger et al. 1993). It is a rapid-onset, short-acting drug marketed as a hypnotic. In multicenter trials, zolpidem was at least as effective as triazolam (Halcion) in treating insomnia in elderly subjects (Maczaj 1993). Adverse effects of BZDs in the elderly are of particular concern, but zolpidem's effects on memory, postural sway, and psychomotor performance appear to be no greater than triazolam's (Hanly and Powles 1993). Despite the greater receptor specificity of zolpidem, it appears to have no significant benefits over the BZDs.

Doses may begin at 5 mg at bedtime and increase to 10 mg, but a beginning dose as low as 2.5 mg may be preferable in elderly patients. Although there is some evidence that zolpidem has a lower risk of tolerance and dependence than other hypnotics, clinical wisdom suggests avoiding long-term use of drugs in this class.

Benzodiazepines

This class contains the drugs most widely used to treat anxiety. Indeed, the BZDs have at times been the most widely prescribed drugs in the national pharmacopoeia. They are extraordinarily safe, with a high therapeutic index and low lethality in overdose when taken alone. They are most useful in the acute management of anxiety, and it is for this indication that most data exist. Currently, 14 BZDs are available on the U.S. market. Although these differ in speed of onset, half-life, metabolic pathways, indications, and liability for abuse, they all have in common four pharmacological effects: anxiolysis, sedation, centrally mediated muscle relaxation, and elevation of seizure threshold. Adverse effects include interference with motor and cognitive functions. Some of the BZDs are marketed as hypnotics (flurazepam, temazepam, triazolam, estazolam, and quazepam), and the rest are marketed for anxiolysis or for parenteral use during surgical or invasive medical procedures. The differences between those marketed as hypnotics and as anxiolytics are somewhat arbitrary but involve half-life and speed of onset. Among the BZDs, there are also other differences in indications. Clonazepam and alprazolam are clearly efficacious in panic disorder, whereas the antipanic effects of the others are less securely established (see Chapter 2). Clonazepam is effective in treating SP and in controlling manic symptoms, and all BZDs will relieve symptoms of anxiety and cross-cover ethanol or barbiturate withdrawal.

BZDs exert their effects by binding to receptors on a macromolecular complex that also includes receptors for GABA and for barbiturates, as well as a chloride ion channel. GABA is a generally inhibitory neurotransmitter that binds to a receptor on this complex with the result that the chloride channel opens and the neuron becomes more polarized and therefore less likely to fire. The binding of BZDs allosterically enhances the action of GABA (Nutt 1990).

In animal models, chronic dosing with BZDs results in downregulation of BZD receptors that follows the same time course as that of tolerance to ataxic effects (Miller et al. 1988a). Tolerance also develops to sedation but not to anxiolysis (Rickels and Schweizer 1990). Although tolerance to the anxiolytic effects does not seem to occur, anxiety is one of several symptoms seen in BZD discontinuation even after only a few weeks of treatment. The higher the dosage and the longer the period of exposure, the more significant the withdrawal symptoms, with seizures and/or delirium constituting the most serious possibilities. Liability for withdrawal symptoms also depends on drug half-life, with shorter-acting BZDs more likely to cause such symptoms than longer-acting ones.

The BZDs share some common structural elements but differ in others. The categorization presented in this section is based on these structural differences, but a detailed explanation of the terminology is beyond the scope of this chapter. The *2-keto* BZDs include diazepam (Valium), chlordiazepoxide (Librium), prazepam (Centrax), clorazepate (Tranxene), halazepam (Paxipam), and flurazepam (Dalmane). All of these agents are oxidatively metabolized in the liver, and their elimination includes metabolites that are themselves active. As a result, the effective half-lives of these drugs, taking into account those of their active metabolites, range from 30 to 200 hours and may be even further increased in the elderly or in people with diminished hepatic function. Quazepam (Doral) is similar in this regard but has a *2-thio* rather than a 2-keto group. Prazepam and clorazepate are considered *prodrugs* in that they themselves are not pharmacologically active, but their efficacy depends on their conversion into active metabolites. The *3-hydroxy* BZDs include lorazepam (Ativan), oxazepam (Serax), and temazepam (Restoril). These agents are biotransformed by glucuronidation and then excreted renally. There are no active metabolites, so half-lives are between 10 and 30 hours and metabolism is less impaired by hepatic dysfunction. The *triazolo* BZDs include triazolam (Halcion), alprazolam (Xanax), and estazolam (ProSom). They are oxidized before glucuronidation but possess no significant active metabolites. Half-lives range from 2–3 hours for triazolam to 10–14 hours for estazolam. The *2-nitro* BZD clonazepam (Klonopin) has a long half-life, ranging between 18 and 50 hours, but no active metabolites.

These differences in metabolism and half-life are important because drugs without active metabolites are safer for patients with liver dysfunction. On the other hand, drugs with slowly eliminated active metabolites tend to produce milder withdrawal syndromes because those metabolites linger, producing a "self-tapering" effect. BZDs differ, too, in rates of absorption from the gastrointestinal tract. Diazepam, lorazepam, triazolam, and estazolam are the most quickly absorbed, a factor that affects their usefulness as acute anxiolytics or hypnotics. Anterograde amnesia, however, is more frequently experienced with the faster-absorbed drugs.

The chief advantages of the BZDs are their safety and efficacy. Their disadvantages are that they are CE drugs and can cause anterograde amnesia (Kanno et al. 1993; Mejo 1992; Shader and Greenblatt 1983), either of which effects can theoretically interfere with CBT. In addition, there is a liability for abuse that is low in the general population, but significant among people with a history of substance dependence (Ciraulo et al. 1988). Table 1–7 lists benzodiazepines currently available in the United States.

Beta-Adrenergic Antagonists

"Beta-blockers" have found their most frequent psychiatric applications in the treatment of performance anxiety and in the alleviation of the restlessness that can be an early adverse effect of SSRIs. They are antagonists at beta-adrenergic receptors and are marketed primarily for use in the treatment of hypertension and some cardiac conditions. Their advantages include low abuse liability and little or no effect on memory and psychomotor performance (Betts et al. 1985; Greenblatt et al. 1993) The beta-blockers are CE drugs and so theoretically may interfere with CBT. Adverse effects include cardiac conduction delay, exacerbation or precipitation of congestive heart failure or asthma, impotence, fatigue, depression, and elevation of blood glucose levels by inhibiting insulin release. These effects are unlikely to occur when the drugs are used only on an occasional basis, but even occasional use is relatively contraindicated in persons with asthma, heart blocks, and low cardiac output states.

Many beta-adrenergic antagonists are available on the U.S. market. They differ in half-life, relative selectivity for subtypes of beta-adrenergic receptors, and lipid solubility. The latter property

Table 1–7. Benzodiazepines

Type	Generic name	Trade name	Relative potency (mg to produce equivalent effect)	Effective half-life (including effects of active metabolites)
7-nitro (metabolites are not active)	Clonazepam	Klonopin	0.25	Long
2-keto (where desmethyl-diazepam is persistent active metabolite)	Chlordiazepoxide	Librium	10	Long
	Diazepam	Valium	6	Long
	Clorazepate	Tranxene	7.5	Long
	Prazepam	Centrax	10	Long
	Halazepam	Paxipam	20	Long
(where N-desalkyl-flurazepam is a persistent active metabolite)	Flurazepam	Dalmane	30	Long
2-thione (where N-desalkyl-flurazepam is a persistent active metabolite)	Quazepam	Doral	6	Long

3-hydroxy (no long-lasting active metabolites)	Lorazepam	Ativan	1	Intermediate
	Oxazepam	Serax	15	Intermediate
	Temazepam	Restoril	30	Intermediate
Triazolo (no long-lasting active metabolites)	Alprazolam	Xanax	0.5	Intermediate
	Triazolam	Halcion	0.25	Short
	Estazolam	Prosom	1	Intermediate
Imidazo	Midazolam (only a parenteral form is available)	Versed		Short

Note. Many of these agents are available generically.

influences how readily a drug can enter the brain, although whether beta-adrenergic blockade–induced anxiolysis is centrally or peripherally mediated is still uncertain. Beta-adrenergic receptors located on the heart are of the $beta_1$ subtype, whereas those on pulmonary bronchi are of the $beta_2$ subtype. There are more $beta_1$ receptors in the brain, and some evidence supports the idea that blockade at the $beta_1$ subtype is more important for anxiolysis (Lader 1990). Atenolol (Tenormin) and metoprolol (Lopressor) are relatively more selective for $beta_1$ receptors and have the advantage of being less likely to cause bronchospasm. Propranolol (Inderal) and nadolol (Corgard) are not selective as regards receptor subtype. Within the $beta_1$-selective group, atenolol is longer acting than metoprolol and in the nonselective group, nadolol is longer acting than propranolol. Table 1–8 lists some of the beta-adrenergic blockers currently available in the United States.

Neuroleptics

Neuroleptics are primarily used in treating the psychoses, including those associated with mood disorders, but these drugs also have anxiolytic properties. All neuroleptics are dopamine receptor antagonists and two, clozapine and risperidone, also block serotonergic receptors. Trifluoperazine (Stelazine) has been granted an FDA indication for the treatment of nonpsychotic anxiety, al-

Table 1–8.   Beta blockers (selective listing)

Generic name	Trade name	Selectivity	Half-life (hours)
Propranolol	Inderal (short-acting)	No	3–6
Atenolol	Tenormin (long-acting)	$Beta_1$	6–9
Nadolol	Corgard (long-acting)	No	14–24
Metoprolol	Lopressor (short-acting)	$Beta_1$	3–4

Note.   These agents are also available generically.

though the other neuroleptics have also been used for their sedative or anxiolytic effects. The neuroleptics would rarely be a first-line choice in the treatment of anxiety, however, because of their many potential adverse effects such as postural hypotension, cardiac conduction delay, effects on motor pathways, and the potentially irreversible adverse effect of tardive dyskinesia. Their chief advantage is the potential for achieving a response in patients whose anxiety is refractory to other treatments. In addition, their abuse liability is low. Table 1–9 lists some of the neuroleptics currently available in the United States.

Prebenzodiazepine Anxiolytics

This group encompasses a wide range of chemical types and is not discussed in detail here because the agents included are seldom a preferred treatment for anxiety disorders. None of the prebenzodiazepine anxiolytics offers a specific effect that other, safer drugs lack. Although this category of drugs will not be further described here, Table 1–10 provides a selective listing of the prebenzodiazepine anxiolytics for interested readers.

Table 1–9.   Neuroleptics (selective listing)

Generic name	Trade name	Dose range for anxiolysis (mg/day)	Potency
Trifluoperazine	Stelazine	1–6	High[*]
Fluphenazine	Prolixin	1–4	High
Perphenazine	Trilafon	4–16	Medium
Chlorpromazine	Thorazine	25–400	Low
Thioridazine	Mellaril	25–400	Low

Note.   These agents are also available generically. *Trifluoperazine is the only neuroleptic with a U.S. Food and Drug Administration (FDA) indication for treatment of anxiety.

Table 1–10. Prebenzodiazepine anxiolytics (selective listing)

Type	Generic name	Trade name
Barbiturates (introduced during early 1900s)	Amobarbital	Amytal
	Butabarbital	Buticaps, Butisol
	Mephobarbital	Mebaral
	Pentobarbital	Nembutal
	Phenobarbital	Luminal
	Secobarbital	Seconal
	Secobarbital with amobarbital	Tuinal
Structural relatives of barbiturates	Glutethimide	Doriden
	Methyprylon	Nodular
Substituted diols, aldehydes, alcohols (introduced in 1950s)	Meprobamate	Equanil, Miltown
	Tybamate	Tybatran, Solacen
	Chloral hydrate	Noctec
	Ethchlorvynol	Placidyl
	Ethinamate	Valmid
Other	Chlormezanone	Trancopal (more common as muscle relaxant)

▐ Anxiolytic Pharmacotherapy in Pregnant Women

No medication is considered to be entirely without risk during pregnancy. Although many of the psychotropic drugs have not definitively been associated with fetal malformations (lithium carbonate is an important exception), ethical problems obviously make it difficult to design a relevant controlled study. Consequently, no psychotropic medication is labeled as indisputably safe in pregnancy.

For some patients, however, the risk of not treating an anxiety disorder exceeds that associated with pharmacotherapy. The risk of relapse of an anxiety disorder is not reduced during pregnancy or the postpartum period and may be increased. Severe untreated anxiety disorders can affect the risk of miscarriage, produce intolerable suffering for the mother, and potentially alter early mother-infant relationships in negative ways. Morbidity from untreated anxiety, moreover, might prevent some women who wish to have children from becoming pregnant. In general, the threshold for pharmacotherapeutic intervention during pregnancy should be elevated but not absolute, and should take into account that some women may reasonably choose to receive pharmacotherapy for a disorder that is debilitating and even potentially life-threatening. When feasible, of course, nonpharmacological therapies should be carefully considered before recommending pharmacotherapy to a woman who is pregnant or who wishes soon to become pregnant.

The use of medications during the first trimester has been considered especially risky because it is during that period that the fetus's organ systems begin to differentiate. It is still somewhat controversial whether BZDs can cause cleft palate if prescribed during the first trimester; recent evidence points away from that conclusion (Bergman et al. 1992; Rosenberg et al. 1983). A syndrome of neurodevelopmental delay has been described in children of mothers using BZDs during pregnancy (Laegreid et al. 1992), however, although this could be the result of comorbid conditions in the women taking BZDs. Abundant animal data do suggest that function at the $GABA_A$ receptor complex is altered in the offspring of animals treated with BZDs during pregnancy (Miller et al. 1989). Such changes could perhaps alter neural development in ways that are not obvious at birth. This question awaits further study, and until the issue is clarified, it is most prudent to avoid BZDs at least during the first trimester of pregnancy. The second and third trimesters are considered safer but may not be completely free of risk, because neural development continues throughout all trimesters and even following birth. No convincing evidence in human populations indicates that BZDs interfere with this process.

No definitive evidence supports an association of TCAs with fetal malformations. One recent study, however, suggested a possible small increase in the rates of miscarriage among women taking TCAs or fluoxetine (Pastuszak et al. 1993). This trend may have been due to the drugs or to other factors associated with the conditions for which they were prescribed. Consequently, antidepressants appear to be the preferred agents for treating anxiety during pregnancy when pharmacotherapy has been appropriately chosen. If TCAs are to be used, changes in physiology during pregnancy may require dosage increases of 1.3 to 2 times the original dose to maintain appropriate serum levels (Wisner et al. 1993).

▋ Issues of Drug Dependency

Barbiturates have a very high potential for abuse, BZDs less so, and dependency is the least to be feared with buspirone, antidepressants, beta-blockers, neuroleptics, or antihistamines. Among the BZDs, risk for abuse and dependence varies. Alprazolam, diazepam, triazolam, and lorazepam appear to pose the greatest risk and chlordiazepoxide, oxazepam, and clorazepate the least (Ciraulo et al. 1991). All persons treated continuously with BZDs for more than a few weeks at a time will become physiologically dependent, but this is not to be confused with abuse. The potential for BZD abuse is higher in persons with a history of substance abuse (Ciraulo et al. 1988) than in those who have never abused substances, and seems related in part to the specific medication's speed of penetration into the central nervous system.

A clinical issue often of even greater importance than liability for developing a drug dependency syndrome in the DSM-IV sense is the fear some patients develop of being unable to function without a medication. For those people who can be treated with nonpharmacological therapies such as CBT, either alone or with initial pharmacotherapy, such treatment is often the superior choice. Some patients, however, will not respond to these forms of treatment and may even require somatic treatment of prolonged duration. With these patients, periodic tapering of the medication and reassessment are recommended to determine whether there continues to be a need for pharmacotherapy. In my experience, initial clarity about the need for this periodic reassessment, combined with a flexible approach to the tapering process, ultimately supports patients' attempts to discontinue pharmacotherapy in a more satisfactory way.

■ Conclusions

The combined use of somatic and psychosocial treatments offers the opportunity for some patients to pursue psychosocial treatment more successfully following an initial trial of pharmacotherapy. Other patients may prefer pharmacotherapy alone and may require medication for extended periods of time, even for the remainder of their lives. Although prolonged pharmacotherapy and drug dependence may seem undesirable, their consequences are often less destructive than the symptoms of severe and untreated anxiety disorders. Despite the prejudicial beliefs of many health care providers and members of the general public, prolonged pharmacotherapy should not be assumed to represent either incompetence on the part of the clinician or moral weakness on the part of the patient. The only way to discover which outcome is most appropriate for a specific patient is for patient and clinician to try different approaches, as clinically appropriate, often in an integrated collaboration among providers of different treatment approaches.

■ References

Agras WS: Treatment of social phobias. J Clin Psychiatry 51:52–58, 1990

American Psychiatric Association: Diagnostic and Statistical Manual of Mental Disorders, 3rd Edition. Washington, DC, American Psychiatric Association, 1980

American Psychiatric Association: Diagnostic and Statistical Manual of Mental Disorders, 3rd Edition, Revised. Washington, DC, American Psychiatric Association, 1987

American Psychiatric Association: Diagnostic and Statistical Manual of Mental Disorders, 4th Edition. Washington, DC, American Psychiatric Association, 1994

Baxter LR, Schwartz JM, Bergman KS, et al: Caudate glucose metabolic rate changes with both drug and behavior therapy for obsessive-compulsive disorder. Arch Gen Psychiatry 49:681–689, 1992

Bergman U, Rosa FW, Baum C, et al: Effects of exposure to benzodiazepine during fetal life. Lancet 340:694–696, 1992

Betts TA, Knight R, Crowe A, et al: Effect of beta-blockers on psychomotor performance in normal volunteers. Eur J Clin Pharmacol 28 (suppl):39–49, 1985

Biederman J, Jellinek MS: Resistance to the anti-anxiety effect of buspirone in patients with a history of benzodiazepine use (letter). N Engl J Med 314:719–720, 1986

Biederman J, Rosenbaum JF, Hirshfeld DR, et al: Psychiatric correlates of behavioral inhibition in young children of parents with and without psychiatric disorders. Arch Gen Psychiatry 47:21–26, 1990

Black B, Tancer ME: Fluoxetine for the treatment of social phobia (letter). J Clin Psychopharmacol 12:293–295, 1992

Blazer D, Hughes D, George LK: Stressful life events and the onset of a generalized anxiety syndrome. Am J Psychiatry 144:1178–1183, 1987

Bourdon KH, Boyd JH, Rae DS, et al: Gender differences in phobias: results of the ECA community survey. Journal of Anxiety Disorders 2:227–241, 1988

Brantigan CO, Brantigan TA, Joseph N: The effect of beta blockade on stage fright: a controlled study. Rocky Mountain Medical Journal 76:227–233, 1979

Brantigan CO, Brantigan TA, Joseph N: Effect of beta blockade and beta stimulation on stage fright. Am J Med 72:88–94, 1982

Brawman MO, Lydiard RB, Emmanuel N, et al: Psychiatric co-morbidity in patients with generalized anxiety disorder. Am J Psychiatry 150:1216–1218, 1993

Briggs NC, Jefferson JW, Koenecke FH: Tranylcypromine addiction: a case report and review. J Clin Psychiatry 51:426–429, 1990

Caron C, Rutter M: Comorbidity in child psychopathology: concepts, issues and research strategies. J Child Psychol Psychiatry 32:1063–1080, 1991

Ciraulo DA, Sands BF, Shader RI: Critical review of liability for benzodiazepine abuse among alcoholics. Am J Psychiatry 145:1501–1506, 1988

Ciraulo DA, Sands BF, Shader RI, et al: Anxiolytics, in Clinical Manual of Chemical Dependence. Edited by Ciraulo DA, Shader RI. Washington, DC, American Psychiatric Press, 1991, pp 135–186

Clark DB, Agras WS: The assessment and treatment of performance anxiety in musicians. Am J Psychiatry 148:598–605, 1991

Clary C, Mandos LA, Schweizer E: Results of a brief survey on the prescribing practices for monoamine oxidase inhibitor antidepressants. J Clin Psychiatry 51:226–231, 1990

Crewe HK, Lennard MS, Tucker GT, et al: The effect of selective serotonin reuptake inhibitors on cytochrome P4502D6 (CYP2D6) activity in human liver microsomes. Br J Clin Pharmacol 34:262–265, 1992

Czepowicz VD, Johnson MR, Emmanuel NP, et al: Sertraline in social phobia (NR95), in New Research Program and Abstracts: American Psychiatric Association, 150th Annual Meeting, Philadelphia, PA, May 21–26, 1994. Washington, DC, American Psychiatric Association, 1994, p 79

Da Prada M, Kettler R, Keller HH, et al: Short-lasting and reversible inhibition of monoamine oxidase-A by moclobemide. Acta Psychiatr Scand Suppl 360:103–105, 1990

Davidson JRT, Ford SM, Smith RD, et al: Long-term treatment of social phobia with clonazepam. J Clin Psychiatry 52 (11, suppl):16–20, 1991

DiNardo P, Moras K, Barlow DH, et al: Reliability of DSM-III-R anxiety disorder categories: using the Anxiety Disorders Interview Schedule—Revised (ADIS-R). Arch Gen Psychiatry 50:251–256, 1993

Dingemanse J: An update of recent moclobemide interaction data. Int Clin Psychopharmacol 7:167–180, 1993

Durham RC, Allan T: Psychological treatment of generalized anxiety disorder: a review of the clinical significance of results in outcome studies since 1980. Br J Psychiatry 163:19–26, 1993

Faigel HC: The effect of beta blockade on stress-induced cognitive dysfunction in adolescents. Clin Pediatr (Phila) 30:441–445, 1991

Feighner JP: Buspirone in the long-term treatment of generalized anxiety disorder. J Clin Psychiatry 48 (12, suppl):3–6, 1987

Feighner JP, Merideth CH, Hendrickson GA: A double-blind comparison of buspirone and diazepam in outpatients with generalized anxiety disorder. J Clin Psychiatry 43:103–108, 1982

Fishbein M, Middlestadt SE, Ottati V, et al: Medical problems among ICSOM musicians: overview of a national survey. Medical Problems of Performing Artists 3:1–8, 1988

Fyer AJ, Mannuzza S, Chapman TF, et al: A direct interview family study of social phobia. Arch Gen Psychiatry 50:286–293, 1993

Galpern WR, Lumpkin M, Greenblatt DJ, et al: The effect of anxiolytic drugs on memory in anxious subjects. Psychopharmacol Ser 6:128–139, 1988

Gammans RE, Stringfellow JC, Hvizdos AJ, et al: Use of buspirone in patients with generalized anxiety disorder and coexisting depressive symptoms: a meta-analysis of eight randomized, controlled studies. Neuropsychobiology 25:193–201, 1992

Gates GA, Saegert J, Wilson N, et al: Effect of beta blockade on singing performance. Ann Otol Rhinol Laryngol 94 (6 pt 2):570–574, 1985

Gelernter CS, Uhde TW, Cimbolic P, et al: Cognitive-behavioral and pharmacological treatments of social phobia. Arch Gen Psychiatry 48:938–944, 1991

Goldman RG, McGrath PJ, Stewart JW, et al: Does antidepressant treatment change personality? (NR384), in New Research Program and Abstracts: American Psychiatric Association, 150th Annual Meeting, Philadelphia, PA, May 21–26, 1994. Washington, DC, American Psychiatric Association, 1994, p 157

Greenblatt DJ, Scavone JM, Harmatz JS, et al: Cognitive effects of beta-adrenergic antagonists after single doses: pharmacokinetics and pharmacodynamics of propranolol, atenolol, lorazepam, and placebo. Clin Pharmacol Ther 53:577–584, 1993

Grillon C, Buchsbaum MS: EEG topography of response to visual stimuli in generalized anxiety disorder. Electroencephalogr Clin Neurophysiol 66:337–348, 1987

Hanly P, Powles P: Comparison of the effects of zolpidem and triazolam on memory functions, psychomotor performances, and postural sway in healthy subjects. J Clin Psychopharmacol 13:100–106, 1993

Heimberg RG, Beecker RE, Goldfinger K, et al: Treatment of social phobia by exposure, cognitive restructuring, and homework assignments. J Nerv Ment Dis 173:236–245, 1985

Heimberg RG, Hope DA, Dodge CS, et al: DSM-III-R subtypes of social phobia: comparison of generalized social phobics and public speaking phobics. J Nerv Ment Dis 178:172–179, 1990

Heinrich K, Lehman E: Low dose neuroleptic anxiolysis in anxiety states. Prog Neuropsychopharmacol Biol Psychiatry 16:136–143, 1991

Hoehn-Saric R, McLeod DR, Zimmerli WD: Differential effects of alprazolam and imipramine in generalized anxiety disorder: somatic versus psychic symptoms. J Clin Psychiatry 49:293–301, 1988

Hymowitz P, Frances A, Jacobsberg LB, et al: Neuroleptic treatment of schizotypal personality disorders. Compr Psychiatry 27:267–271, 1986

James I, Savage I: Beneficial effect of nadolol on anxiety-induced disturbances of performance in musicians: a comparison with diazepam and placebo. Am Heart J 108 (4 pt 2):1150–1155, 1984

Jenike MA, Surman OS, Cassem NH, et al: Monoamine oxidase inhibitors in obsessive-compulsive disorder. J Clin Psychiatry 44:131–132, 1983

Kagan J, Reznick JS, Snidman N: Biological basis of childhood shyness. Science 240:167–171, 1988

Kanno O, Watanabe H, Kazamatsuri H: Amnestic effects of triazolam and other hypnotics. Prog Neuropsychopharmacol Biol Psychiatry 17:407–413, 1993

Kendler KS, Neale MC, Kessler RC, et al: Generalized anxiety disorder in women: a population-based twin study. Arch Gen Psychiatry 49:267–272, 1992a

Kendler KS, Neale MC, Kessler RC, et al: The genetic epidemiology of phobias in women: the interrelationship of agoraphobia, social phobia, situational phobia, and simple phobia. Arch Gen Psychiatry 49:273–281, 1992b

Kendler KS, Neale MC, Kessler RC, et al: Major depression and generalized anxiety disorder: same genes, (partly) different environments? Arch Gen Psychiatry 49:716–722, 1992c

Lader M: Beta$_2$-adrenoceptor antagonism in anxiety. Eur Neuropsychopharmacol 1:75–77, 1990

Laegreid L, Hagberg G, Lundberg A: Neurodevelopment in late infancy after prenatal exposure to benzodiazepines: a prospective study. Neuropediatrics 23:60–67, 1992

Lahmeyer HW, Reynolds CF, Kupfer DJ, et al: Biologic markers in borderline personality disorder: a review. J Clin Psychiatry 50:217–225, 1989

Liebowitz MR, Fyer AJ, Gorman JM, et al: phenelzine in social phobia. J Clin Psychopharmacol 6:93–98, 1986

Liebowitz MR, Schneier FR, Hollander E, et al: Treatment of social phobia with drugs other than benzodiazepines. J Clin Psychiatry 52 (11, suppl):10–15, 1991

Liebowitz MR, Schneier F, Campeas R, et al: phenelzine vs. atenolol in social phobia: a placebo-controlled comparison. Arch Gen Psychiatry 49:290–300, 1992

Lindsay WR, Gamsu CV, McLaughlin E, et al: A controlled trial of treatments for generalized anxiety disorder. Br J Clin Psychol 26:3–15, 1987

Maczaj M: Multicenter, double-blind, controlled comparison of zolpidem and triazolam in elderly patients with insomnia. Clin Ther 15:127–136, 1993

Mann JJ, Aarons SF, Wilner PJ, et al: A controlled study of the antidepressant efficacy and side effects of (–)deprenyl: a selective monoamine oxidase inhibitor. Arch Gen Psychiatry 46:45–50, 1989

Marks IM: Comparative studies on benzodiazepines and psychotherapies. Encephale 9 (4 suppl 2):23B–30B, 1983

Martins EA, Pigott TA, Bernstein S, et al: Sertraline pharmacotherapy in patients with social phobia (NR60), in New Research Program and Abstracts: American Psychiatric Association, 150th Annual Meeting, Philadelphia, PA, May 21–26, 1994. Washington, DC, American Psychiatric Association, 1994, p 69

Mejo SL: Anterograde amnesia linked to benzodiazepines. Nurse Pract 17:49–50, 1992

Mendels J, Krajewski TF, Huffer V, et al: Effective short-term treatment of generalized anxiety disorder with trifluoperazine. J Clin Psychiatry 47:170–174, 1986

Miller LG, Kastin AJ: Persistent elevation in $GABA_A$ receptor subunit mRNAs following social stress. Brain Res Bull 26:809–812, 1991

Miller LG, Greenblatt DJ, Barnhill JG, et al: The dexamethasone suppression test in generalized anxiety disorder. Br J Psychiatry 149:320–322, 1986

Miller LG, Greenblatt DJ, Barnhill JG, et al: Chronic benzodiazepine administration, I: tolerance is associated with benzodiazepine receptor downregulation and decreased gamma-aminobutyric acid-A receptor function. J Pharmacol Exp Ther 246:170–176, 1988a

Miller LG, Galpern WR, Byrnes JJ, et al: Differential modulation of benzodiazepine receptor binding by ethanol in LS and SS mice. Pharmacol Biochem Behav 29:471–477, 1988b

Miller LG, Chesley S, Galpern WR, et al: Prenatal lorazepam administration is associated with GABA$_A$ receptor alterations in late embryonic and mature chicks. Neurotoxicology 10:517–522, 1989

Munjack DJ, Baltazar PL, Bohn PB, et al: Clonazepam in the treatment of social phobia: a pilot study. J Clin Psychiatry 51 (5, suppl):35–40; discussion 50–53, 1990

Nestadt G, Romanoski AJ, Samuels JF, et al: The relationship between personality and DSM-III Axis I disorders in the population: results from an epidemiological survey. Am J Psychiatry 149:1228–1233, 1992

Nies A: Differential response patterns to MAO inhibitors and tricyclics. J Clin Psychiatry 45 (7 pt 2):70–77, 1984

Nutt DJ: The pharmacology of human anxiety. Pharmacol Ther 47:233–266, 1990

Papp LA, Gorman JM, Liebowitz MR, et al: Epinephrine infusions in patients with social phobia. Am J Psychiatry 145:733–736, 1988

Pastuszak A, Schick-Boschetto B, Zuber C, et al: Pregnancy outcome following first-trimester exposure to fluoxetine (Prozac). JAMA 269:2246–2248, 1993

Paykel ES, White JL: Clinical psychopharmacology of beta-adrenoceptor antagonism in treatment of anxiety. Annals of the Academy of Medicine, Singapore 20:43–45, 1991

Pollack MH, Rosenbaum JF: Management of antidepressant-induced side effects: a practical guide for the clinician. J Clin Psychiatry 48:3–8, 1987

Potts NL, Davidson JRT, Krishnan KR, et al: Levels of urinary free cortisol in social phobia. J Clin Psychiatry 52:41–42, 1991

Proctor RC: Results with fluphenazine in anxiety and tension. Diseases of the Nervous System 21:283–285, 1960

Quitkin F, Rifkin A, Klein DF: Monoamine oxidase inhibitors: a review of antidepressant effectiveness. Arch Gen Psychiatry 36:749–760, 1979

Rabkin J, Quitkin F, Harrison W, et al: Adverse reactions to monoamine oxidase inhibitors, I: a comparative study. J Clin Psychopharmacol 4:270–278, 1984

Rapaport M: The epidemiology of social phobia. Symposium presented at the New Clinical Drug Evaluation Unit (NCDEU) Meeting, Marco Island, Florida, May 1994

Regier DA, Boyd JH, Burke JD, et al: One-month prevalence of mental disorders in the United States: based on five Epidemiologic Catchment Area sites. Arch Gen Psychiatry 45:977–986, 1988

Reich J, Noyes RJ, Yates W: Alprazolam treatment of avoidant personality traits in social phobic patients. J Clin Psychiatry 50:91–95, 1989

Reich J, Yates W: Family history of psychiatric disorders in social phobia. Compr Psychiatry 29:72–75, 1988a

Reich J, Yates W: A pilot study of treatment of social phobia with alprazolam. Am J Psychiatry 145:590–594, 1988b

Reiter SR, Pollack MH, Rosenbaum JF, et al: Clonazepam for the treatment of social phobia. J Clin Psychiatry 51:470–472, 1990

Rickels K, Schweizer E: The clinical course and long-term management of generalized anxiety disorder. J Clin Psychopharmacol 10 (suppl):101S–110S, 1990

Rickels K, Schweizer E: The treatment of generalized anxiety disorder in patients with depressive symptomatology. J Clin Psychiatry 54 (1, suppl):20–23, 1993

Rickels K, Schweizer E, Csanalosi I, et al: Long-term treatment of anxiety and risk of withdrawal: prospective comparison of clorazepate and buspirone. Arch Gen Psychiatry 45:444–450, 1988

Roger M, Attali P, Coquelin JP: Regional differences in the enhancement by GABA of [^{3}H]zolpidem binding to omega$_1$ sites in rat brain membranes and sections. Brain Res 600:134–140, 1993

Rosenbaum JF: Treatment of outpatients with desipramine. J Clin Psychiatry 45 (10 sec 2):225–226, 1984

Rosenbaum JF, Biederman J, Hirshfeld DR, et al: Behavioral inhibition in children: a possible precursor to panic disorder or social phobia. J Clin Psychiatry 52 (11, suppl):5–9, 1991

Rosenberg L, Mitchell AA, Parsells JL, et al: Lack of relation of oral clefts to diazepam use during pregnancy. N Eng J Med 309:1281–1285, 1983

Schneier FR, Johnson J, Hornig CD, et al: Social phobia: comorbidity in an epidemiologic sample. Arch Gen Psychiatry 49:282–288, 1992

Schweizer E, Rickels K: Failure of buspirone to manage benzodiazepine withdrawal. Am J Psychiatry 143:1590–1592, 1986

Shader RI, Greenblatt DJ: Triazolam and anterograde amnesia: all is not well in the Z-zone (editorial). J Clin Psychopharmacol 3:273, 1983

Sheehan DV, Ballenger J, Jacobsen G: Treatment of endogenous anxiety with phobic, hysterical, and hypochondriacal symptoms. Arch Gen Psychiatry 37:51–59, 1980

Siever LJ, Davis KL: A psychobiological perspective on the personality disorders. Am J Psychiatry 148:1647–1658, 1991

Stein MB, Tancer ME, Gelernter CS, et al: Major depression in patients with social phobia. Am J Psychiatry 147:637–639, 1990

Stein MB, Tancer ME, Uhde TW: Heart rate and plasma norepinephrine responsivity to orthostatic challenge in anxiety disorders: comparison of patients with panic disorder and social phobia and normal control subjects. Arch Gen Psychiatry 49:311–317, 1992

Stewart JW, Walsh BT, Wright L, et al: An open trial of MAO inhibitors in bulimia. J Clin Psychiatry 45:217–219, 1984

Tancer ME, Stein MB, Gelernter CS, et al: The hypothalamic-pituitary-thyroid axis in social phobia. Am J Psychiatry 147:929–933, 1990

Tellegen A, Lykken OT, Bouchard TJ, et al: Personality similarity in twins reared apart. J Pers Soc Psychol 54:1031–1039, 1988

Tipton KF, O'Carroll A, Mantle TJ, et al: Factors involved in the selective inhibition of monoamine oxidase. Mod Probl Pharmacopsychiatry 19:15–30, 1983

Tyrer P, Seivewright N, Murphy S, et al: The Nottingham study of neurotic disorder: comparison of drug and psychological treatments. Lancet 2:235–240, 1988

Uhde TW, Tancer ME, Black B, et al: Phenomenology and neurobiology of social phobia: comparison with panic disorder. J Clin Psychiatry 52 (11, suppl):31–40, 1991

Uhlenhuth EH, Balter MB, Mellinger GD, et al: Symptom check-list syndromes in the general population: correlations with psychotherapeutic drug use. Arch Gen Psychiatry 40:1167–1173, 1983

Wisner KL, Perel JM, Wheeler SB: Tricyclic dose requirements across pregnancy. Am J Psychiatry 150:1541–1542, 1993

Wittchen HU, Essau CA: Fluoxetine efficacy in social phobia. J Clin Psychiatry 54:27–32, 1993

Wittchen HU, Zhao S, Kessler RC, et al: DSM-III-R generalized anxiety disorder in the national comorbidity survey. Arch Gen Psychiatry 51:355–364, 1994

Wu D, Otton SV, Sproule BA, et al: Differential effects of the anxiolytic drugs, diazepam and buspirone, on memory function. Br J Clin Pharmacol 23:207–211, 1987

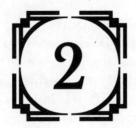

Panic Disorder: Pharmacotherapy in Integrative Treatment

Christine Pfaelzer, M.D., M.P.H.,
James M. Ellison, M.D., M.P.H., and
Sabrina Popp, M.D.

Panic disorder is estimated to have a lifetime prevalence of 1.5% in the U.S. adult population (Weissman 1994). Its peak onset is in young adulthood, after which it typically follows a chronic, relapsing course (Keller and Hanks 1993). The disorder is roughly twice as prevalent among women as among men (Regier et al. 1988). Although panic disorder often causes immense distress, functional impairment, and demoralization, the prognosis made possible by current treatment approaches is excellent. The necessity for appropriate and timely treatment is further underscored by evidence that panic disorder sufferers frequently find their way into medical settings, where they consume unnecessary diagnostic and treatment services at an excessive rate (Katon et al. 1990). Further-

more, panic disorder is associated with an increased rate of suicidal ideation and attempts (Weissman 1994), although suicidality
may be associated primarily with the panic attack state (Korn et al.
1994) or be at least partially attributable to past or current comorbid depression (Cox et al. 1994). In this chapter we first review
current pharmacotherapeutic approaches to the treatment of
panic disorder. We then illustrate some clinical issues relevant to
an integrated treatment approach to complement the discussion
offered in Chapter 3.

▌ Definition of Panic Disorder

"Nervousness" is a very common condition, affecting as many as
one-quarter of the large community samples of U.S. adults surveyed in the Epidemiologic Catchment Area study (Weissman
1994). The recent National Comorbidity Survey (Eaton et al.
1994) reported that 15% of the U.S. population have experienced
a panic attack at some time. To meet the full criteria for the diagnosis of panic disorder, an individual must experience full-blown,
discrete attacks of anxiety, or at least 1 month of persistent fear of
another attack following one or more attacks. These may begin
within the context of an upsetting situation but evolve into spontaneous, unexpected episodes. According to DSM-III-R (American Psychiatric Association 1987), such an attack consists of at
least four of a cluster of physical symptoms that represents the
consequences of autonomic nervous system hyperactivity. Shortness of breath (dyspnea), dizziness or faintness, palpitations, accelerated heart rate, and sweating are the most common examples of
attack symptoms, although trembling, choking, nausea, numb-
ness, flushes, chills, or chest discomfort are also frequently experienced (American Psychiatric Association 1987). These physical
symptoms are characteristically accompanied by depersonalization, derealization, or fears of dying, going crazy, or losing control. Typically, panic symptoms escalate in intensity and decline to
a residual level of anxiety within a 20-minute interval. Although

they often occur two to three times each week, their rate can vary. DSM-IV (American Psychiatric Association 1994) shifts the emphasis of the diagnostic criteria for panic disorder in three important ways. First, the actual number of attacks is less emphasized. Next, the importance of anticipatory anxiety is underscored by requiring for this diagnosis the presence of persistent concern, worry, or behavioral changes related to the attacks. Finally, panic disorder is not diagnosed if another anxiety disorder can better account for the presence of panic attacks.

For many panic disorder patients, the fear of an impending panic attack produces even more distress and disability than the attacks themselves. Between attacks, such patients experience increasing anticipatory anxiety characterized by inhibition, fear of medical illness, role dysfunction, and feelings of helplessness and/or humiliation. The estimated one-third of panic disorder sufferers who develop agoraphobia (Weissman 1994) find themselves preoccupied with intense fears of being in places from which escape may be problematic or help difficult to obtain in the event of a panic attack. Bridges, trains, busses, and crowded areas are among the many sites that become associated with fear and avoidance. Ultimately, an agoraphobic individual may fear to venture unaccompanied from the relative safety of home.

Assigning a diagnosis of panic disorder implies that the reasonable likelihood of a medical disorder underlying the anxiety symptoms has been considered and rejected. Because symptoms identical to those of panic can also be produced by any of a wide variety of substance abuse, endocrinological, metabolic, neurological, infectious, or toxic disorders, an appropriate effort must be made to discover these potential causes before a definitive diagnosis can be reached. In particular, patients should be questioned about their use of caffeine, prescribed medications, and substances of abuse, since these agents may produce physical symptoms identical to those of panic disorder or may complicate the treatment of panic symptoms. In the initial workup of a panic disorder patient, it is often prudent to perform or request a general medical screening that includes a careful inquiry about drug use, or even a toxic screen; a complete blood count; liver and thyroid function tests; and an electrocardiogram (Coplan et al. 1993; see also Chapter 8).

■ Pharmacotherapeutic Goals and Agents

The efficacy of pharmacotherapy in treating panic disorder has been demonstrated in many careful investigations. We recently combined for meta-analysis the results of 31 placebo-controlled, randomized, double-blind studies that used alprazolam or imipramine and found that between-study analyses could be performed only with respect to the two measures employed nearly universally: panic attack frequency counts and Hamilton Anxiety Scale (Hamilton 1959) scores. On the basis of these measures, alprazolam and imipramine were each found clearly superior to placebo (C. Pfaelzer and J. M. Ellison, unpublished data, January 1994). As reviewed below, many additional medications appear to have valid roles in the treatment of panic disorder.

The particular aspects of panic disorder that are most responsive to pharmacotherapy alone remain a topic of debate. Medications are of proven usefulness in quickly decreasing the intensity and frequency of panic attacks, but appear less effective in treating avoidant or anticipatory anxiety. Currently published studies make it difficult to be certain about this conclusion, however, and leave relatively unexplored the question of medication effects on secondary impairment of social or occupational functioning.

Before prescribing medication, a clinician should attempt to understand the full extent of a specific patient's difficulties, including associated symptoms such as phobic avoidance; comorbid disorders such as substance abuse, other Axis I disorders, or personality disorders; and impairment of social and occupational role functions. This information facilitates appropriate and comprehensive treatment planning. In addition, the prescribing clinician will want to consider pharmacotherapy's place within the larger treatment context. As will be illustrated in the case vignettes that appear later in this chapter, medications can be combined with cognitive-behavioral psychotherapy in a variety of ways. With some patients, the initial use of medications allows for rapid symptom control, supporting the patient's functioning while cognitive-behavioral treatment is initiated. With others, a synergistic relationship develops between pharmacotherapy and psychotherapy when the two are offered concurrently. Whatever the sequence of treatments, patients should be appropriately educated about the available options so that they can make informed choices.

Four classes of drugs currently are considered to possess proven efficacy in treating panic disorder: the benzodiazepines, the tricyclic antidepressants (TCAs), the monoamine oxidase inhibitors (MAOIs), and, more recently, the selective serotonin reuptake inhibitors (SSRIs). Anticonvulsants such as carbamazepine and valproate, beta-blocking antiadrenergic agents such as propranolol, and azapirones such as buspirone have also been suggested to be effective, but their use is less fully supported by controlled research. Because each medication class has therapeutic advantages and disadvantages, the selection of a particular drug is based on an individualized evaluation of the patient.

Many clinicians consider the benzodiazepines a first-line choice in the acute treatment of panic disorder. Among this class of agents, alprazolam has been the most extensively studied (Ballenger et al. 1988; Cross-National Collaborative Panic Study 1992; Deltito et al. 1991; Lesser et al. 1988; Lydiard et al. 1992; Munjack et al. 1989; Swinson et al. 1987; Taylor et al. 1990). Clonazepam, better tolerated than alprazolam by some patients because it is longer acting, has also garnered much support for use as an antipanic agent (Svebak et al. 1990; Tesar et al. 1991). Other benzodiazepines that have been used and studied with varying degrees of success include diazepam, adinazolam (not yet available in the United States), and lorazepam (Noyes et al. 1984, Pyke and Greenberg 1989; Schweizer et al. 1990; Sheehan 1987). The benzodiazepines have been shown to significantly decrease the frequency and intensity of panic attacks. To a considerable extent, they also reduce anticipatory anxiety and may have antiphobic properties (Deltito et al. 1991; Lydiard et al. 1992; Munjack et al. 1989; Swinson et al. 1987). Benzodiazepines are particularly valued for their rapid onset of action and minimal adverse effects. Patients often experience relief of symptoms within hours to days, in contrast to the week or more that may be required to achieve the full effect of treatment with agents from other medication classes.

In treatment of panic disorder patients, benzodiazepine doses begin low and are titrated upward to reach a maximally therapeutic level while minimizing side effects. Alprazolam, which is metabolized relatively quickly, is often given three to four times a day to reduce fluctuations in serum level. Less-frequent dosing, for some patients, is associated with increased anxiety prior to the next dose (Herman et al. 1987), although dosing at more frequent intervals can impair compliance. A typical therapeutic total daily dosage of alprazolam falls between 2 and 8 mg/day. The latest dose is given as close to bedtime as possible to minimize early-morning rebound anxiety symptoms (Coplan et al. 1993). In a recent report by Greenblatt and associates (1993), a plasma alprazolam level of 20 ng/day was identified as a therapeutic threshold. Increased rates of remission and decreased symptoms correlated with levels between 20 and 39 ng/ml. Above 39 ng/ml, no additional clinical benefits were seen.

The production of tolerance (the need for increasing dosages to achieve an equivalent effect) and physical dependence (the occurrence of physical symptoms upon drug withdrawal) are the benzodiazepines' most distinct disadvantages. Other benzodiazepine drawbacks include excessive daytime drowsiness (their most frequently reported side effect), impaired coordination, interdose anxiety, and rebound anxiety that can follow treatment discontinuation. After extended benzodiazepine use, withdrawal symptoms can be intense. Abrupt discontinuation of benzodiazepine treatment may pose physical danger as a result of withdrawal effects.

A longer-term drawback of benzodiazepine treatment is its association with a high postdiscontinuation relapse rate. Some studies have reported recurrence of panic attacks or other withdrawal symptoms in as many as 70% to 89% of patients being tapered off alprazolam (Dupont and Pecknold 1985; Fyer et al. 1987; Noyes et al. 1991). This complication can be mitigated to some extent by using longer-acting benzodiazepines such as clonazepam (Herman et al. 1987) or adjunctive cognitive-behavior therapy (Otto et al. 1992).

The TCAs are another frequently used class of antipanic medications. Imipramine, the most thoroughly studied TCA, has been found efficacious in several placebo-controlled, double-blind studies (e.g., Cross-National Collaborative Panic Study 1992; Deltito et al. 1991; Modigh et al. 1992; Robinson et al. 1989; Sheehan et al. 1988; Taylor et al. 1990). Desipramine, clomipramine, amitriptyline, and nortriptyline have to lesser extents been used and studied (Modigh et al. 1992; Lydiard and Ballenger 1987), although their efficacy may well be similar to that of imipramine. TCAs are often a first-line choice for panic disorder or may be used after failure of a benzodiazepine regimen. The antidepressant effects of TCAs make them more effective than benzodiazepines for patients with comorbid depression.

TCAs affect panic attacks similarly to the benzodiazepines, but may take a few weeks to achieve their maximal effect. Some studies have attributed greater antiphobic effects to imipramine than to the benzodiazepines (Cross-National Collaborative Panic Study 1992; Lydiard and Ballenger 1987; Sheehan et al. 1980; Zitrin et al. 1980, 1983). The fact that TCAs can be given in a single daily dose confers a distinct potential advantage in terms of compliance. Unfortunately, many patients complain of their side effects, which can be more prominent than those of the benzodiazepines (Cross-National Collaborative Panic Study 1992); these effects include dry mouth, blurred vision, constipation, tachycardia, hypotension, sedation, weight gain, sexual dysfunction, and changes in cardiac conduction. As with the benzodiazepines, TCAs are initially prescribed in small doses that are gradually increased, with attention to the development of side effects. Patients who do not respond at 200 mg/day of imipramine, or its equivalent, should have their dosages increased to 300 mg/day if the side effects are tolerable. Plasma tricyclic level determinations can help guide pharmacotherapy in patients who experience severe side effects at low doses or appear unresponsive at standard doses. Some patients, whose low plasma medication levels may reveal them to be rapid metabolizers, will require doses in excess of 300 mg/day (Coplan et al. 1993).

Discontinuation of TCAs is less likely to produce unpleasant symptoms than is discontinuation of benzodiazepines. Symptom recurrence, however, is common. Noyes and colleagues (1989), for example, found that half of the panic disorder patients who had responded successfully to a tricyclic antidepressant relapsed upon its discontinuation during the subsequent 1–4 years of follow-up included in their naturalistic study. Another study found a 75% relapse rate among patients previously responsive to imipramine. The use of a half-dose maintenance protocol was associated with better outcome on measures including panic severity and phobic anxiety/avoidance (Mavissakalian and Perel 1992).

Another antidepressant class, the MAOIs, has been very successful in the treatment of panic disorder, although it is not clear whether the efficacy of the MAOIs outweighs their potentially serious side effects. MAOIs now tend to be used after patients have failed courses of several other medications. The beneficial effects of phenelzine, isocarboxazid (no longer available in the United States), and tranylcypromine have been elucidated in a few well-constructed studies that revealed these agents to have particular efficacy in alleviating panic attacks and associated depressive symptoms, with less pronounced effects on measures of phobic avoidance or anticipatory anxiety (Buigues and Vallejo 1987; Quitkin et al. 1990).

The development of a hypertensive crisis that results from the interaction of MAOIs with certain foods or medications is the most serious potential side effect of this drug class. Patients must be educated about the necessary dietary and medication restrictions. They also need to be advised that the occurrence of headache or lightheadedness may indicate postural hypotension, another common and potentially dangerous side effect of this class of drugs. In addition, hepatocellular damage occasionally results from MAOI use. Because of these potential effects on the body, prescribing clinicians monitor both blood pressure and liver enzymes of patients undergoing treatment with MAOIs.

The efficacies of the SSRI antidepressants in treating panic disorder are still being explored, and the small number of published placebo-controlled trials limits the generalizability of current results. Fluoxetine and fluvoxamine are the two most widely studied of these agents so far (Clark and Jacob 1994; Den Boer and Westenberg 1988, 1990; Gorman et al. 1987; Hoehn-Saric et al. 1993; Schneier et al. 1990). Sertraline, paroxetine, venlafaxine, and nefazodone each await further study. The SSRIs' low incidence of side effects makes them particularly attractive treatment agents. Sedation and anticholinergic effects, so troublesome with TCAs and MAOIs, are rare with SSRIs. SSRIs, however, may require a number of weeks to be fully effective, and they do sometimes produce unpleasant side effects, including gastrointestinal upset, headache, restlessness, sedation, or sexual dysfunction. In addition, a thought-provoking anecdotal report noted the development of apathy and/or indifference on SSRIs (Hoehn-Saric et al. 1990). As with the other classes of drugs, it would be premature to draw conclusions about what specific factors of panic disorder the SSRIs most affect, but their therapeutic efficacies appear comparable to those of other medication classes in reducing panic attack frequency (Den Boer and Westenberg 1988; Gorman et al. 1987; Hoehn-Saric et al. 1993; Schneier et al. 1990). Preliminary data suggest a less dramatic effect of SSRIs on global improvement measures (Den Boer and Westenberg 1990). As with the other classes of drugs, doses should be started low, even as low as 1.25–5 mg/day for fluoxetine, and titrated gradually upward to avoid compliance-impairing side effects (Gorman et al. 1987; Schneier et al. 1990).

Scattered evidence supports the usefulness of other drug classes in the treatment of panic disorder. Two antiepileptic medications, carbamazepine (Keck et al. 1992) and valproate (Woodman and Noyes 1994), have been shown to have beneficial effects. Propranolol, a beta-blocker, has been proposed to have a role in the treatment of panic disorder but has been reported to be less efficacious than the benzodiazepines (Munjack et al. 1989; Noyes 1985). Although it achieved results comparable to those of imipramine in one study that used low imipramine doses (Munjack et al. 1985), propranolol is believed, in contrast to imipramine, to lack the capacity to block lactate-induced panic attacks (Gorman et al. 1982). In one well-designed study, buspirone proved superior to placebo in reducing frequency of panic attacks (Robinson et al. 1989), although other studies suggest that buspirone occasionally induces attacks in panic disorder patients (Chignon et al. 1994).

Many questions remain to be answered regarding the pharmacotherapy of panic disorder. High dropout rates, lack of standardized outcome measures, substance abuse, and surreptitious drug use are just a few of the problems that have limited the generalizability of available research findings. Further studies are needed to elucidate, for instance, which aspects of panic disorder should prompt a clinician to resort to pharmacotherapy rather than psychotherapy or should suggest combined treatment. In addition, there are as yet no standard recommendations regarding pretreatment medical evaluation, initial choice of antipanic medication, length of pharmacotherapy, or process of medication discontinuation. The role of integrated treatment approaches in panic disorder is addressed later in this chapter.

▌ Approaches to Pharmacotherapy-Resistant Panic Disorder Patients

The effects of medication are rarely entirely satisfactory. Some patients fail to benefit, while others are helped only to a limited degree or tolerate treatment poorly because of adverse effects. In many instances, the pharmacologically oriented clinician may elect to recommend adjunctive cognitive-behavior therapy, but the addition of another treatment approach should not replace or curtail the clinician's effort to find the most appropriate pharmacotherapeutic regimen.

Addressing pharmacotherapy-resistant cases of panic disorder, Coplan and co-workers (1993) recently reported a three-step approach. First, they recommended discerning whether the medication was properly prescribed and dispensed. Inadequate dosage, inadequate dosage frequency (as discussed previously with the benzodiazepines), and insufficient treatment duration are common reasons for treatment failure. Inadequate treatment can result from clinician factors, such as failure to consider the possibility of rapid metabolism, or from patient factors, such as poor compliance.

Second, Coplan and colleagues suggested a reexamination of the patient for comorbid mental disorders that could interfere with the effectiveness of treatment. Substance abuse, depression, or personality disorders are common comorbid findings in panic disorder patients. At least one study has correlated poorer outcomes with the presence of certain personality disorders (Reich 1988), and several studies have pointed to worse outcomes for panic disorder patients with untreated comorbid depression (Lesser et al. 1988; Reich 1988). Another potential confounder of treatment is patients' undisclosed supplementation of therapy with nonprescribed medications. Using controlled observation, investigators have discovered the presence of unexpected benzodiazepines in the plasma of 25%–35% of their subjects (Clark et al. 1990; Lydiard et al. 1992).

Finally, it is often worthwhile to reassess a treatment-resistant patient for evidence of underlying medical disorders. When seemingly appropriate treatment fails to produce a positive response, the possibility of organic illness should be reconsidered. A more complete cardiac, neurological, or endocrinological workup may be indicated, depending on the patient's specific symptoms (see also Chapter 8).

For reasons that often remain speculative, some patients respond better to particular drugs, or drug combinations, than to others. When one drug or drug class proves ineffective, therefore, it is often worthwhile to consider other agents, alone or in combination. Failing this, the clinician may want to reconsider combining pharmacotherapy with cognitive-behavior therapy. This sequence is not presented as a standard, because there are also compelling reasons to *begin* treatment with cognitive-behavior therapy (see Chapter 3). Some of the benefits and hazards of a combined treatment approach are discussed in more detail in the following section, supplemented with illustrative clinical vignettes.

▌ Combining Pharmacotherapy With Psychotherapy for Panic Disorder

Treatment approaches are combined in the belief that a more positive effect will be achieved than is attainable with a single modality. This advantage can be conferred through greater effects on the same symptoms (*additive* or *synergistic* effects) or through effects on differing clusters of symptoms (*complementary* effects). In some cases, providing two treatment approaches can produce undesirable interference with one or both treatments' effectiveness. Studies of panic disorder that have addressed these issues have primarily examined combinations of cognitive-behavioral psychotherapy and a tricyclic antidepressant or a benzodiazepine.

A pioneering study examined the combined effects of imipramine and exposure therapy on panic disorder patients and demonstrated additive effects after 14 weeks of the two therapies on measures of global improvement, phobia, and panic as compared with exposure therapy plus placebo (Zitrin et al. 1980). In another study, Marks and colleagues (1983) found imipramine to enhance the effects of exposure therapy on several indices, though the additive benefits from imipramine appeared to be time limited. In a review of existing studies on combined treatment, Mavissakalian (1989) suggested that the combination of imipramine with cognitive-behavior therapy actually had an additive effect, specifically on phobic symptoms.

Shear (1991) has discussed some of the many possible interactions of combined treatment approaches. Among these, some clinicians emphasize the particular effectiveness of medications in reducing panic attack frequency, whereas cognitive-behavior therapy may have greater value in reducing anticipatory anxiety and general disability (Nagy et al. 1989, 1993). Rapidity of symptom alleviation provides another area of complementarity. As illustrated in the following vignette, pharmacotherapy can provide rapid relief, facilitating a patient's later entry into an adjunctive cognitive-behavioral treatment:

Mr. A, a 41-year-old married man, had a long history (> 5 years) of panic symptoms. He had been reluctant to seek treatment because of fears that "people would think I'm crazy," but his attacks had begun to have a very negative impact on his work performance, resulting even in absences from work. He wanted "something to work quickly" because of concerns about his job. Mr. A responded to clonazepam, 1 mg tid, with a reduction of attacks and a return to more normal activity. He felt sedated on this dose and described "having less of the drive that I need"; however, attempts to lower the dose resulted in a return of symptoms.

Mr. A was prescribed desipramine in gradually increasing doses and clonazepam was discontinued. Again, his panic was alleviated but he developed significant side effects, including severe dry mouth (an intolerable problem in view of the public speaking required by his job), a weight gain of 15 pounds, and decreased sexual potency. At that point, Mr. A agreed to a referral to a cognitive-behavioral therapist. He was gradually taken off medication, and he worked regularly with the cognitive-behavioral therapist over the next 3 months. During this interval, he initially had some panic episodes, but with the passage of time he was able to control and then alleviate his symptoms. Mr. A continued in treatment for 1 year to work on his panic symptoms and other issues. He required no further medications.

The complementarity of a combined treatment approach can also allow a patient to achieve more comprehensive relief from symptoms. Although either medications or psychotherapy can have broader effects, it is often the case that medications relieve panic attack symptoms while adjunctive cognitive-behavioral treatment alleviates dysfunction associated with anticipatory and phobic anxiety, as illustrated in the following case example:

Ms. B, a 33-year-old single mother, had severe panic symptoms that led her to seek treatment. She reported three to four attacks daily, with severe physical symptoms that included severe shaking, palpitations, shortness of breath, near–fainting spells, and severe nausea with vomiting. She had become quite agoraphobic as well, was unable to travel alone, and could no longer do grocery shopping or meet her daughter at school to bring her home.

Ms. B was tried on a variety of medications, including nortriptyline, phenelzine, alprazolam, imipramine, fluoxetine, clonazepam, and combinations of these. Although she improved significantly from her baseline, she continued to have daily attacks and remained significantly agoraphobic.

At the time of referral to a cognitive-behavioral therapist, Ms. B was taking imipramine 200 mg at bedtime and clonazepam 1 mg tid. She was still experiencing three to four attacks per week, although their intensity had decreased. A decision was made by the cognitive-behavioral therapist and the pharmacotherapist to maintain Ms. B's medications during psychotherapy.

The cognitive-behavioral treatment allowed Ms. B to address her remaining symptoms and to learn more effective means for coping with them. Gradually, she became able to resume her shopping, meet her daughter at school, travel alone (except on the subway), and return to social activities. In Ms. B's words, "These treatments have given me back my life and my ability to play with my daughter and be a good mother."

Thorough psychoeducational preparation of the patient is an important aspect of combining treatment approaches. A patient's unrealistic expectations or limited understanding of the relative roles of psychotherapy and pharmacotherapy can lead to premature termination of one or the other approach. The following example demonstrates how such inadequate understanding of treatment components helped to impede one patient's recovery:

Mr. C, a 28-year-old man who had been in cognitive-behavioral treatment for 3 months, reported moderate success with the treatment but still had episodes of what he called "significant anxiety" and wanted medication as an adjunct to his current treatment. He had discussed this wish with his psychotherapist, who encouraged him to obtain a medication consultation. Mr. C described episodes of still becoming quite anxious and sweating but not going on to full panic attacks because of his ability to control further symptom development through the techniques he had learned. He was started on clonazepam 0.5 mg bid, which produced full resolution of his symptoms.

Soon afterward, Mr. C decided to terminate his cognitive-behavior therapy because "It's just stupid exercises; I can do them at home," and "I feel so much better on the medications, I don't need it." Although he was encouraged to continue in treatment by the cognitive-behavioral therapist and the pharmacotherapist, he nonetheless terminated cognitive-behavioral treatment the following week. About 1 month later, Mr. C noticed a return of his anxiety symptoms and requested an increase in medications. When questioned about his exercises, he stated, "They were boring; I haven't been doing them." Further medication increases brought about side effects that interfered with his work, yet did not fully control his symptoms. Mr. C then agreed to resume cognitive-behavioral treatment, stating, "I guess there's no quick fix; I guess I need both." With combined treatment, his symptoms soon resolved once again and he was able to decrease the doses of his medications.

Termination of pharmacotherapy often is made easier by concurrent psychotherapy that has allowed a patient to learn and practice cognitive and behavioral skills that reduce the likelihood of symptomatic relapse. Discontinuation of antipanic medication—particularly of benzodiazepines—can present great difficulties for patients. Even when the medication is slowly tapered, the onset of withdrawal symptoms is often experienced as a recurrence of panic attacks, resulting in anxious reluctance to part with medications (Herman et al. 1987; Noyes et al. 1991). Evidence from the literature supports a role for cognitive-behavior therapy with patients unable to tolerate the effects of a benzodiazepine taper. Otto and co-workers (1992) reported from an ongoing study that 8 of 10 patients using adjunctive cognitive-behavior therapy to facilitate benzodiazepine taper were able to successfully discontinue their medication, whereas only 3 of 11 patients not using adjunctive cognitive-behavior therapy were able to do so.

▌ Providing Pharmacotherapy Within a Psychotherapeutic Relationship

Participation in combined therapy, despite its potential in many cases for producing a superior clinical outcome, is often rejected as a treatment option. Some patients resist the increased initial investment of time or money, while others choose to try pharmacotherapy alone on the basis of their preference for a biomedical explanation of their symptoms. It is particularly important, with such patients, to recognize that a psychotherapeutic *relationship* can enhance the effectiveness of pharmacotherapy even in the absence of more extensive psychotherapeutic *treatment*. Beitman (1991) has proposed a stage-oriented paradigm that alerts clinicians to psychotherapeutic considerations relevant to each of the four phases of psychotherapy. In Table 2–1, we have adapted and simplified his paradigm for application to the treatment of an anxiety disorder. Four temporal stages of pharmacotherapy are identified with respect to goals, techniques, resistance, and transference/countertransference issues. The principles identified are relevant to the psychodynamic aspects of pharmacotherapy, whether provided by, or in collaboration with, a psychotherapist.

▌ Conclusions

In this chapter we have summarized the current state of pharmacotherapy of panic disorder and reviewed some benefits and hazards of combining pharmacotherapy with cognitive-behavioral psychotherapy. The panic disorder literature contains only a limited number of well-designed trials examining the comparative efficacies of medications with or without concurrent psychotherapy. High dropout rates, insufficient numbers of control subjects, surreptitious adjunctive drug use, and lack of standardized anxiety indices remain significant methodological limitations of currently published studies—and, consequently, barriers to the determination of a definitive treatment approach to this disorder. It is likely

Table 2–1. Stages of pharmacotherapy delivered within a psychotherapeutic relationship

	Stage 1: Assessment and engagement	Stage 2: Identification of symptom patterns	Stage 3: Symptom response	Stage 4: Termination or maintenance
Goals	Develop therapeutic alliance; agree upon treatment contract	Formulate syndromal diagnosis; identify target symptoms	Alleviate or eliminate target symptoms; reduce associated disability	Separate efficiently or make smooth transition to maintenance phase
Techniques	Empathic evaluation, psychoeducation, informed consent	Use of both open-ended and specific syndrome-oriented questions; use of additional informants when appropriate	Choice of effective medication, appropriate dosage and schedule; monitoring of symptoms, side effects, and compliance	Ongoing preparation of patient from beginning of treatment; terms acceptable to patient and therapist
Resistance	Reluctance to accept pharmacotherapy may indicate resistance	Patterns of compliance and side effects may reveal and clarify resistance	Poor compliance or excessive side effects may represent resistance to change	Recurrence of symptoms or side effects may indicate need for further preparation prior to termination

(continued)

Table 2–1. Stages of pharmacotherapy delivered within a psychotherapeutic relationship (*continued*)

	Stage 1: Assessment and engagement	Stage 2: Identification of symptom patterns	Stage 3: Symptom response	Stage 4: Termination or maintenance
Transference to pharmacotherapist	Attend to patient's view of pharmacotherapist as excessively good or bad, powerful or ineffective, respectful or threatening	Pattern of response to symptom change, side effects, or alterations in treatment may reflect transference issues	Transference changes during course of treatment may accompany or signal progress or setback	Unwillingness to relinquish or impulsive rejection of medications may reflect need to address transference
Countertransference	Inappropriate choice to provide or withhold pharmacotherapy suggests interfering countertransference	Incorrect target symptom identification, diagnosis, or treatment recommendations suggest interfering countertransference	Prescribing behavior aimed inappropriately at expediting or prolonging treatment may reflect interfering countertransference	Premature termination or excessively prolonged maintenance phase may reflect interfering countertransference

Source. Adapted from Beitman 1991, p. 22.

that considerations of clinical effectiveness as well as cost-benefit issues will confirm the advantages of combining treatment approaches for many patients, and so we await the results of further studies that address this question.

▌ References

American Psychiatric Association: Diagnostic and Statistical Manual of Mental Disorders, 3rd Edition, Revised. Washington, DC, American Psychiatric Association, 1987

American Psychiatric Association: Diagnostic and Statistical Manual of Mental Disorders, 4th Edition. Washington, DC, American Psychiatric Association, 1994

Ballenger JC, Burrows GD, Dupont RL, et al: Alprazolam in panic disorder and agoraphobia: results from a multicenter trial. Arch Gen Psychiatry 45:413–422, 1988

Beitman BD: Medications during psychotherapy: case studies of the reciprocal relationship between psychotherapy process and medication use, in Integrating Pharmacotherapy and Psychotherapy. Edited by Beitman BD, Klerman GL. Washington, DC, American Psychiatric Press, 1991, pp 21–43

Buigues J, Vallejo J: Therapeutic response to phenelzine in patients with panic disorder and agoraphobia with panic attacks. J Clin Psychiatry 48:55–59, 1987

Chignon J-M, Martin PM, Lepine J-P: Buspirone induced panic: Possible role of 1-(2-pyrimidinyl) piperazine (NR230), in New Research Program and Abstracts: American Psychiatric Association, 150th Annual Meeting, Philadelphia, PA, May 21–26, 1994. Washington, DC, American Psychiatric Association, 1994, p 115

Clark DB, Jacob RG: A double-blind placebo-controlled pilot study of fluoxetine for panic disorder (NR243), in New Research Program and Abstracts: American Psychiatric Association, 150th Annual Meeting, Philadelphia, PA, May 21–26, 1994. Washington, DC, American Psychiatric Association, 1994, pp 118–119

Clark DB, Taylor CB, Roth WT, et al: Surreptitious drug use by patients in a panic disorder study. Am J Psychiatry 147:507–509, 1990

Coplan JD, Tiffon L, Gorman JM: Therapeutic strategies for the patient with treatment-resistant anxiety. J Clin Psychiatry 54 (5, suppl):69–74,1993

Cox BJ, Direnfeld BA, Swinson RP, et al: Suicidal ideation and suicide attempts in panic disorder and social phobia. Am J Psychiatry 151:882–887, 1994

Cross-National Collaborative Panic Study, Second Phase Investigators: Drug treatment of panic disorder. Br J Psychiatry 160:191–202, 1992

Deltito JA, Argyle N, Klerman G, et al: Patients with panic disorder unaccompanied by depression improve with alprazolam and imipramine treatment. J Clin Psychiatry 52:121–127, 1991

Den Boer JA, Westenberg HGM: Effect of a serotonin and noradrenaline uptake inhibitor in panic disorder: a double-blind comparative study with fluvoxamine and maprotiline. Int Clin Psychopharmacol 3:59–74, 1988

Den Boer JA, Westenberg HGM: Serotonin function in panic disorder: a double-blind placebo-controlled study with fluvoxamine and ritanserin. Psychopharmacology 102:85–94, 1990

Dupont RL, Pecknold JC: Alprazolam withdrawal in panic disorder patients (NR81), in New Research Program and Abstracts: American Psychiatric Association, 138th Annual Meeting, Dallas, TX, May 18–24, 1985. Washington, DC, American Psychiatric Association, 1985, p 54

Eaton WW, Kessler RC, Wittchen HU, et al: Panic and panic disorder in the United States. Am J Psychiatry 151:413–420, 1994

Fyer AJ, Liebowitz MR, Gorman JM, et al: Discontinuation of alprazolam treatment in panic patients. Am J Psychiatry 144:303–308, 1987

Gorman JM, Levy GF, Liebowitz MR, et al: Effect of acute beta-adrenergic blockade on lactate-induced panic. Arch Gen Psychiatry 40:1079–1082, 1982

Gorman JM, Liebowitz MR, Fyer AJ, et al: An open trial of fluoxetine in the treatment of panic attacks. J Clin Psychopharmacol 7:329–332, 1987

Greenblatt DJ, Harmatz JS, Shader RI: Plasma alprazolam concentrations: relation to efficacy and side effects in the treatment of panic disorder. Arch Gen Psychiatry 50:715–722, 1993

Hamilton M: The assessment of anxiety states by rating. Br J Med Psychol 32:50–55, 1959

Herman JB, Brotman AW, Rosenbaum JF: Rebound anxiety in panic disorder patients treated with shorter-acting benzodiazepines. J Clin Psychiatry 48 (10, suppl):22–26, 1987

Hoehn-Saric R, McLeod DR, Hipsley PA: Effect of fluvoxamine on panic disorder. J Clin Psychopharmacol 13:321–326, 1993

Hoehn-Saric R, Lipsey JR, McLeod DR: Apathy and indifference in patients on fluvoxamine and fluoxetine. J Clin Psychopharmacol 10:343–345, 1990

Katon W, Von Korff M, Lin E, et al: Distressed high utilizers of medical care: DSM-III-R diagnoses and treatment needs. Gen Hosp Psychiatry 12:355–362, 1990

Keck PE, McElroy SL, Friedman LM: Valproate and carbamazepine in the treatment of panic and posttraumatic stress disorders, withdrawal states, and behavioral dyscontrol syndromes. J Clin Psychopharmacol 12 (1 suppl):36S–41S, 1992

Keller MB, Hanks DL: Course and outcome in panic disorder. Prog Neuropsychopharmacol Biol Psychiatry 17:551–570, 1993

Korn ML, Plutchik R, van Praag H: Panic associated suicide and violence (NR262), in New Research Program and Abstracts: American Psychiatric Association, 150th Annual Meeting, Philadelphia, PA, May 21–26, 1994. Washington, DC, American Psychiatric Association, 1994, pp 123–124

Lesser IM, Rubin RT, Pecknold JC, et al: Secondary depression in panic disorder and agoraphobia. Arch Gen Psychiatry 45:437–443, 1988

Lydiard RB, Ballenger JC: Antidepressants in panic disorder and agoraphobia. J Affect Disord 13:153–168, 1987

Lydiard RB, Lesser IM, Ballenger JC, et al: A fixed-dose study of alprazolam 2 mg, alprazolam 6 mg, and placebo in panic disorder. J Clin Psychiatry 12:96–103, 1992

Marks IM, Gray S, Cohen D, et al: Imipramine and brief therapist-aided exposure in agoraphobics having self-exposure homework. Arch Gen Psychiatry 40:153–162, 1983

Mavissakalian M: Differential effects of imipramine and behavior therapy on panic disorder with agoraphobia. Psychopharmacol Bull 25:27–29, 1989

Mavissakalian M, Perel JM: Clinical experiments in maintenance and discontinuation of imipramine therapy in panic disorder with agoraphobia. Arch Gen Psychiatry 49:318–323, 1992

Modigh K, Westberg P, Eriksson E: Superiority of clomipramine over imipramine in the treatment of panic disorder: a placebo-controlled trial. J Clin Psychopharmacol 12:251–261, 1992

Munjack DJ, Crocker B, Cabe D, et al: Alprazolam, propanolol, and placebo in the treatment of panic disorder and agoraphobia with panic attacks. J Clin Psychopharmacol 9:22–27, 1989

Munjack DJ, Rebal R, Shaner R, et al: Imipramine versus propranolol for the treatment of panic attacks: a pilot study. Compr Psychiatry 26:80–89, 1985

Nagy LM, Krystal JH, Charney DS, et al: Long-term outcome of panic disorder after short-term imipramine and behavioral group treatment: 2.9-year naturalistic follow-up study. J Clin Psychopharmacol 13:16–24, 1993

Nagy LM, Krystal JH, Woods SW, et al: Clinical and medication outcome after short-term alprazolam and behavioral group treatment in panic disorder. Arch Gen Psychiatry 46:993–999, 1989

Noyes R: Beta-adrenergic blocking drugs in anxiety and stress. Psychiatr Clin North Am 8:119–132, 1985

Noyes R, Anderson DJ, Clancy J, et al: Diazepam and propranolol in panic disorder and agoraphobia. Arch Gen Psychiatry 41:287–292, 1984

Noyes R, Garvey MJ, Cook B, et al: Controlled discontinuation of benzodiazepine for patients with panic disorder. Am J Psychiatry 148:517–523, 1991

Noyes R, Garvey MJ, Cook BL, et al: Problems with tricyclic antidepressant use in patients with panic disorder or agoraphobia: results of a naturalistic follow-up study. J Clin Psychiatry 50:163–169, 1989

Otto MW, Pollack MH, Meltzer-Brody S, et al: Cognitive-behavioral therapy for benzodiazepine discontinuation in panic disorder patients. Psychopharmacol Bull 28:123–130, 1992

Pyke RE, Greenberg HS: Double-blind comparison of alprazolam and adinazolam for panic and phobic disorders. J Clin Psychopharmacol 9:15–21, 1989

Quitkin FM, McGrath PJ, Stewart JW, et al: Atypical depression, panic attacks, and response to imipramine and phenelzine: a replication. Arch Gen Psychiatry 47:935–941, 1990

Regier DA, Boyd JH, Burke JD, et al: One-month prevalence of mental disorders in the United States: based on five Epidemiologic Catchment Area sites. Arch Gen Psychiatry 45:977–986, 1988

Reich JH: DSM-III personality disorders and the outcome of treated panic disorder. Am J Psychiatry 145:1149–1152, 1988

Robinson DS, Shrotriya RC, Alms DR, et al: Treatment of panic disorder: nonbenzodiazepine anxiolytics, including buspirone. Psychopharmacol Bull 25:21–26, 1989

Schneier FR, Liebowitz MR, Davies SO, et al: Fluoxetine in panic disorder. J Clin Psychopharmacol 10:119–121, 1990

Schweizer E, Pohl R, Balon R, et al: Lorazepam vs. alprazolam in the treatment of panic disorder. Pharmacopsychiatry 23:90–93, 1990

Shear MK: Panic disorder, in Integrating Pharmacotherapy and Psychotherapy. Edited by Beitman BD, Klerman GL. Washington, DC, American Psychiatric Press, 1991, pp 143–164

Sheehan DV: Benzodiazepines in panic disorder and agoraphobia. J Affect Disord 13:169–181, 1987

Sheehan DV, Ballenger J, Jacobsen G: Treatment of endogenous anxiety with phobic, hysterical, and hypochondriacal symptoms. Arch Gen Psychiatry 37:51–59, 1980

Sheehan DV, Raj AB, Sheehan KH, et al: The relative efficacy of buspirone, imipramine, and placebo in panic disorder: a preliminary report. Pharmacol Biochem Behav 29:815–817, 1988

Svebak S, Cameron A, Levander S: Clonazepam and imipramine in the treatment of panic attacks: a double-blind comparison of efficacy and side effects. J Clin Psychiatry 51 (5, suppl):14–17, 1990

Swinson RP, Pecknold JC, Kuch K: Psychopharmacological treatment of panic disorder and related states: a placebo-controlled study of alprazolam. Prog Neuropsychopharmacol 11:105–113, 1987

Taylor CB, Hayward C, King R, et al: Cardiovascular and symptomatic reduction effects of alprazolam and imipramine in patients with panic disorder: results of a double-blind, placebo-controlled trial. J Clin Psychopharmacol 10:112–118, 1990

Tesar GE, Rosenbaum JF, Pollack MH, et al: Double-blind, placebo-controlled comparison of clonazepam and alprazolam for panic disorder. J Clin Psychiatry 52:69–76, 1991

Weissman MM: Panic disorder: epidemiology and genetics, in Treatment of Panic Disorder: A Consensus Development Conference. Edited by Wolfe BE, Maser JD. Washington, DC, American Psychiatric Press, 1994, pp 31–39

Woodman CL, Noyes R: Panic disorder: treatment with valproate. J Clin Psychiatry 55:134–136, 1994

Zitrin CM, Klein DF, Woerner MG: Treatment of agoraphobia with group exposure in vivo and imipramine. Arch Gen Psychiatry 37:63–72, 1980

Zitrin CM, Klein DF, Woerner MG, et al: Treatment of phobias, I: comparison of imipramine hydrochloride and placebo. Arch Gen Psychiatry 40:125–136, 1983

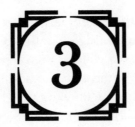

Panic Disorder: Cognitive-Behavioral Treatment and Its Integration With Pharmacotherapy

R. Harris G. McCarter, Ph.D.

———

The efficacies of both pharmacological and cognitive-behavioral treatments for panic disorder are now well established. Luborsky (1993) estimated the success rates at about 80% for cognitive-behavior therapy and 70% for pharmacotherapy. Other recent reviews concur that both treatments are highly effective, with consistently higher rates of response for cognitive-behavioral treatment (Mavissakalian 1991; Michelson and Marchione 1991; Shear 1991). In clini-

I would like to thank Shelley Davis, Ed.D., for her comments on an earlier draft of this chapter.

cal practice, the two treatments are often combined. Empirical studies of treatment combining cognitive-behavioral and pharmacological approaches have yielded mixed results. Some reviews of the literature have suggested that the addition of medication can in some instances impair the effectiveness of cognitive-behavioral treatment (Basoglu 1992). Others, however, have found that the two treatments can be synergistic (Mavissakalian 1991). Perhaps the clearest finding regarding combined treatments is that the addition of cognitive-behavioral interventions can reduce relapse following discontinuation of medication (Michelson and Marchione 1991; Otto et al. 1992, 1993).

Clinical experience with numerous cases suggests that the thoughtful integration of cognitive-behavioral treatment with pharmacotherapy often yields results that neither approach could achieve alone. On the other hand, experience makes it equally clear that when combined treatments are not effectively coordinated, they can work against each other. Written from the perspective of a cognitive-behavior therapist, this chapter describes cognitive-behavioral treatment and reviews issues pertinent to its integration with pharmacotherapy. Its intent is to provide the information that clinicians undertaking combined treatment will need in order to coordinate the combination in an integrated and effective way.

∎ Cognitive-Behavioral Treatment

Several well-designed manuals and self-help books describe cognitive-behavioral treatments of panic disorder (e.g., Babior and Goldman 1990; Barlow and Cerny 1988; Bourne 1990). The best results have been associated with those protocols (e.g., Barlow and Craske 1990, 1994; Craske and Barlow 1993) that include exposure to interoceptive cues (internal sensations that are associated with panic and have become triggers for it). The approach described in this section is most greatly indebted to the protocol developed by Barlow and his associates. The discussion draws primarily on observations made in adapting that protocol to group or individual treatment in an urban hospital behavioral medicine clinic, where the majority of patients carry multiple psychiatric diagnoses and receive concurrent pharmacotherapy. It is noteworthy that this is a very different population from that with which most of the outcome research has been done. As Otto and his associates (1994) have noted, patients with comorbid conditions of a severity commonly seen in clinical practice are systematically excluded from most such studies. It would not be surprising to find that, for multiproblem populations, combined treatment can have a value that the research to date has failed to identify.

A Cognitive-Behavioral Model of Panic Disorder

This treatment approach is based on a model that regards panic disorder as the result of an interaction between neurobiological predisposition and environmental stress. Stressors may be physical, interpersonal, or intrapsychic. Predisposition may begin with excessive inborn reactivity of biological alarm response systems. This inborn reactivity may be modified by subsequent experience, and these modifications may become biologically stable and autonomous. The greater the predisposition, the less stress it takes to evoke traumatic levels of arousal; similarly, with greater stress, less predisposition is required.

This model posits that biological reactivity evolves not only in interaction with environmental stressors but also through interaction with concurrently evolving cognitive, behavioral, and affective processes. In the case of panic disorder, this evolving interactive process results in mounting levels of chronic arousal. Increasingly intense physiological, cognitive, behavioral, and affective reactions take place in response to increasingly subtle stressors. The life events leading up to an initial panic attack will almost always have entailed repeated and substantial stress; however, by the time the attack occurs, chronic arousal and reactivity will often have reached such a pitch that the immediate precipitant goes unrecognized and the attack is subjectively perceived as spontaneous.

The panic state involves the activation of psychophysiological alarm response systems. This activation is designed to signal immediate and intense danger and to prepare the organism to take responsive action. In addition to preparing the organism physiologically, the alarm state also involves activation of the following schemas: 1) cognitive schemas for scanning and meaning-making to identify the danger, 2) affective schemas to motivate the organism with a mounting urge to act in response to that danger once it has been identified, and 3) automatic learning schemas (including but not limited to classical conditioning) to facilitate future identification and avoidance of the danger should it recur.

In the alarm state, all these schemas are activated simultaneously. Once these schemas are activated, moreover, their tendency is to persist until some sort of closure signal is achieved. One type of closure is for physiological, cognitive, affective, and learning schemas to achieve coordination as the organism manages to identify the threat, take effective action, and form associations to facilitate avoidance of the threat in the future. Another is for the panic experience to be recognized as a "false alarm." This, too, involves integration of schemas, as cognitive scanning mechanisms identify the stimulus that triggered the alarm and meaning-making schemas appraise the stimulus as innocuous, thereby activating downregulation of the fight-or-flight response and discharge of tension in a sense of relief. This type of integrated downregulation of alarm response schemas is actually an everyday occurrence—as when, for example, we realize that the police car whose flashing light has appeared behind us intends to pass us by, or that some sound that has startled us is in fact innocuous.

Further study of the mechanisms of false-alarm recognition and downregulation might deepen our understanding of the psychophysiology of panic attacks. It may be, for instance, that false-alarm recognition activates some sort of biological "all clear" mechanism, releasing neurochemicals that neutralize or modify the action of those evoked during the alarm state. An inborn deficiency or stress-induced depletion of alarm-neutralizing neurochemicals or their receptors might be a component of the biological disposition to panic attacks. It is also interesting to consider that the failure of neurobiological closure mechanisms in cognitive scanning for danger may be a variant of a similar inability to achieve closure in checking or grooming schemas that appears to be a component of obsessive-compulsive disorder. The inability to recognize a false alarm may be a biological relative of the inability to "know" that a stove is turned off or that one's hands are clean. My own clinical observations suggest that such closure mechanisms have a biological component, since some patients undergoing pharmacotherapy for obsessive-compulsive disorder have evinced an enhanced capacity for cognitive closure that is seemingly independent of other psychotherapeutic interventions.

One critical feature of a panic attack, then, may be the failure to recognize a false alarm as such. Despite the absence of a "real" danger, cognitive, affective, and learning schemas nonetheless persist. They maintain the person in a state of extreme arousal, terror, and vigilance, all of which are compounded by an intense urge to action. Because there is no identifiable threat, this urge to act is without object or direction, adding elements of frustration, helplessness, and confusion to its already overwhelming intensity. Lacking an appropriate object, the alarm response becomes focused on innocent elements of the internal and external environments. Patients with panic disorder will frequently report how objectively harmless sensations and random aspects of previous panic situations have become associated with catastrophizing cognitions, mistaken conclusions, and avoidant behavior.

Probably because evolution has favored the survival of organisms that could rapidly learn to avoid danger, human beings tend to be equipped with a capacity for one-trial learning with respect to anxiety. This means that the pairing of a particular stimulus with the experience of anxiety need occur only once in order for the stimulus to become a conditioned cue for future anxiety. As a person struggles to make sense of his or her initial panic episode, those aspects of the situation that become a focus of attention may therefore tend to become potential triggers for subsequent panic episodes. In the same way, internal stimuli such as subvocal verbalizations (*self-talk* or *internal dialogue*), mental images, or bodily sensations (*interoceptive cues*) may also become triggers. For example,

I have known patients for whom sitting in a particular type of chair, smelling Chinese food, sneezing, or experiencing an increase in heart rate had become cues for recurrent panic. In each case, the stimulus had been an aspect of the initial panic experience.

Not everyone, however, goes on to develop panic disorder following an initial episode. Meaning-making and learning are critical factors in determining who develops the disorder. Following the first attack, the likelihood of recurrence will depend on the extent to which individuals are alarmed by their panic experience, the degree to which they get caught up in subsequent anxious apprehension and vigilance, and the extent to which external or internal stressors conspire to maintain them in a state of chronic high arousal. Each recurrence tends to further escalate a network of interdependent factors, including predisposing biochemical conditions, physiological and cognitive reactivity, and dread of the panic state itself, thus making subsequent recurrences more likely. Current theory and treatment (e.g., Craske and Barlow 1993; Otto et al. 1994) particularly emphasize the role of the "fear of fear" syndrome in this process. More than any other single factor, the patient's catastrophizing dread of the anxiety state itself is hypothesized to be the driving force that sustains and escalates the disorder.

A factor that further contributes to this escalation of vulnerability is the proliferation and reinforcement of learned cues. With each recurrence, more and more objects, situations, cognitions, and sensations have an opportunity to become associated with panic or to have existing associations strengthened. Thus, patients with panic disorder will frequently describe living in an environment that has become increasingly populated with cues for panic. To the extent that avoidant behavior develops, the person can also become agoraphobic.

Cognitive-Behavioral Treatment of Panic Disorder

Cognitive-behavioral treatment of panic disorder is designed to reverse the resulting destructive positive-feedback loop. The therapy process can be broken down into four main components, which are usually folded into the treatment in roughly the following order: 1) psychoeducation, 2) relaxation/self-soothing, 3) cognitive restructuring, and 4) exposure/desensitization. Furthermore, in some cases there will be a need to work with the family system as well as with the individual patient.

Psychoeducation

The psychoeducational component of treatment provides information. Its goals are to reduce fear and shame, provide a foundation for the development of a new way of viewing the panic experience, empower the panic sufferer, and establish a treatment alliance by offering a model of how and why panic disorder develops. Finally, psychoeducation also makes treatment more acceptable by providing the basis for a mutually agreed-upon treatment plan.

Many persons with panic disorder feel intense shame about the problem. They often suffer in isolation, experiencir.g themselves as uniquely defective and deviant, on a lonely road toward insanity or death. Actually, between 7 and 12 million Americans have been estimated to be agoraphobic (Barlow and Craske 1994). According to data from the National Comorbidity Survey (Eaton et al. 1994), 15% of the U.S. population have experienced a panic attack at some point, and 3% have had an attack within the past month. These data elicit surprised relief from most patients, often freeing them to talk about their experience of deviance and shame. Such a discussion frequently leads to changes in self-perception, especially in a group setting, where the patient is meeting others who describe similar experiences, which gives a human face and palpable reality to the epidemiological findings.

In individual psychotherapy, where this group effect is unavailable, the mere act of reading the diagnostic criteria from the DSM can feel liberating to some patients, providing tangible proof that their experiences conform to a common, expectable, and clinically familiar configuration. On the other hand, some will react in an opposite fashion, taking the existence of a DSM diagnostic description as evidence of how "sick" they are, or taking the clinician's identification of their condition as an attempt to pigeon-hole them with a pathological label. This diversity of possible responses illustrates the importance of tailoring psychoeducation to the needs and vulnerabilities of the patient's self-representing and self-evaluating processes. Psychoeducational information should always be presented with an eye toward the schemas that will be available to assimilate it. In some cases, before sharing information, it may be necessary to prepare the patient for its appropriate reception.

Information on the adaptive function of anxiety and on the physiology of the fight-or-flight response is also useful in reducing both shame and fear. The physical changes and sensations that occur during panic tend to be experienced as a catastrophic, incomprehensible, and possibly deadly breakdown of the body's normal life-support systems. The process becomes far more bearable when its components are understood and placed in the context of a natural, potentially protective coping response whose pathology lies only in its having been activated unnecessarily.

Presentation of this information is generally most helpful when it is integrated with an examination of prior assumptions and beliefs. What meaning has the patient previously attributed to her panic experiences? How has her view of herself been affected? How are these interpretations changing in response to what she is learning in therapy? Such discussion minimizes the extent to which old beliefs may continue to coexist side by side with but unmodified by the new information. The patient's experience of panic is not likely to be instantly and completely transformed by psychoeducation alone; however, psychoeducation provides a foundation for later changes and often does lead to significant relief in its own right.

Psychoeducation should also provide a model of how and why panic disorder and agoraphobia develop and an outline of treatment derived from that model. In the cognitive-behavioral approach to panic, treatment is largely derived from adapting a predetermined protocol to the needs of the individual patient. Compliance and the probability of success will be enhanced if the patient is an informed consumer with an understanding of what he or she is going to be asked to do and why. Psychoeducation is not a matter of pouring information into the ear of a passively receptive patient; rather, it is an interactive and collaborative process.

As treatment progresses beyond psychoeducation, it begins to branch in two directions. The therapist begins to provide the patient with specific tools for coping with anxiety. Simultaneously, patient and therapist begin to collaborate in a process of information gathering through the patient's self-monitoring. For purposes of explication, I first discuss relaxation techniques. Self-monitoring will then be discussed in the subsection on cognitive restructuring.

Relaxation/Self-Soothing

When the therapist introduces relaxation training, the patient is likely to be most interested in the potential use of these techniques to reduce acute distress. Patients will vary in the extent to which they find relaxation techniques helpful in the management of acute anxiety. Of equal importance is the way that the techniques can reduce chronic baseline levels of arousal when they are practiced on a daily basis over a period of weeks. The patient should be informed about both types of benefits and encouraged to invest the time and effort required to achieve the long-term, potentially more significant effects.

A variety of relaxation techniques are available, including progressive muscle relaxation (PMR), diaphragmatic breathing, meditation, guided imagery, hypnosis, and biofeedback. Instructions for PMR and for breathing-based techniques can be found in Barlow and Craske's *Mastery of Your Anxiety and Panic II* (1994). Bourne (1990) provides alternate instructions for these procedures and for imagery-based techniques. Among Western clinical approaches to meditation, Benson's (1975) relaxation response and Kabat-Zinn's (1990) version of mindfulness meditation contain instructions that are easily understood and describe techniques whose efficacy has been validated by extensive research programs. An excellent introduction to the general use of hypnosis can be found in Brown and Fromm's *Hypnotherapy and Hypnoanalysis* (1986); Clarke and Jackson (1983) provide a thorough discussion of the application of hypnosis to the treatment of anxiety disorders. Biofeedback requires substantial hardware and training, and the patient wishing to use it should be referred to a specialist.

Between 50% and 60% of panic disorder patients rate the sensations associated with hyperventilation as being similar to their panic attacks (Craske and Barlow 1993). This may explain why the majority of patients who complete group treatment for panic disorder at The Cambridge Hospital's Behavioral Medicine Program report breathing retraining to be the single most helpful aspect of the treatment. Some, however, find other techniques more helpful. It is my recommendation that patients be encouraged to experiment with a range of techniques, preferably including at least one that addresses breathing, one that addresses muscle tension, one that addresses imagery, and some type of meditation.

There are two reasons for this recommendation. First, it is empowering of and respectful to patients to give them choices. Second, the experience of panic is a systemwide, multidimensional one whose components include changes in muscle tension, in breathing, in the content and organization of imagery and thought, and in self-observation. Most patients will have at least some need for soothing in all these areas and will benefit to some extent from exposure to a corresponding spectrum of techniques. At the same time, patients will differ in their styles and preferences, finding some techniques more relevant and useful than others.

Paradoxical responses to any of the relaxation techniques are possible. In the absence of input from the therapist, such experiences will almost always lead to abandonment of the offending technique; however, most paradoxical responses can be overcome, and it is usually clinically useful to do so. A paradoxical response to a given technique often indicates the degree of reactivity and dysregulation of the specific psychophysiological processes addressed by that technique. If, for example, a man experiences discomfort when asked to attend to his breathing, this may indicate that breathing is an area in which he is in particular need of tools for mastery and self-soothing. A graded-exposure approach to the problematic technique—especially in combination with more comfortable relaxation procedures—will often be effective. A patient who goes into spasm or panic when practicing PMR techniques, for example, may master the procedure by approaching it gradually, beginning with flexion of just a single hand or even a single finger, and flexing only long enough and tightly enough to produce challenging but manageable tension. A similar approach may be taken with any of the other techniques.

When effective, relaxation techniques help place the regulation of arousal under more conscious control. In the process of learning to control breathing or muscle tension, the panic sufferer becomes more aware of these processes and of the routine fluctuations that had previously taken place beyond awareness. A woman who begins to practice PMR may become newly aware of the spontaneous changes in muscle tension that occur throughout the day: how she tenses her shoulders whenever her boss approaches, or how she clenches her jaw whenever she performs a fine motor task. A man who has practiced diaphragmatic breathing may discover that he tends to hold his breath whenever he concentrates, or that he breathes more rapidly when he is under stress. Patients, having noticed these behaviors and being in possession of skills that enable them to respond differently, can begin to consciously modify their responses and to understand and control their experiences in new ways. As they become more mindful, panic sufferers not only begin to have more control over what had previously been unconsciously self-escalating physiological processes but also become more aware of patterns of thought and behavior that can trigger and be triggered by autonomic arousal.

Over time, with regular relaxation practice, arousal is usually reduced. Its components become increasingly differentiated, and the patient's experience of it becomes increasingly organized. In panic disorder, arousal, thought, and behavior tend to fuse into a global, inarticulate, and overwhelming cascade of intense distress whose components are undifferentiated, uncontrolled, and reciprocally exacerbating. With relaxation practice, as arousal decreases and control increases, patients tend to become progressively able to separate the sensations they experience in a given situation from the meaning they attribute to that situation. At lower levels of arousal, they are better able to learn that the *feeling* that something terrible is happening can be experienced even when no actual danger is present. Thus, relaxation training paves the way for cognitive restructuring of the catastrophizing thought processes that tend to escalate and sustain the panic state. Reduced catastrophizing diminishes the psychological suffering associated with the physiological arousal, and as suffering declines, further reciprocal reductions in arousal tend to occur as well. The result is a helpful feedback loop in which learning reduces suffering and reinforces its own effect.

For most patients, the changes brought about by relaxation practice are experienced as achievements of the self, leading to increased feelings of resourcefulness, mastery, self-efficacy, and self-esteem. Furthermore, these relaxation techniques remain a part of a person's repertoire for coping with future stressors. Individuals who experience a return of symptoms upon decreased or discontinued practice usually return to effective levels without a sense of shame or defeat, and a substantial number find the practice (especially of meditation) so rewarding in its own right that they would not give it up even if they felt assured that they would never have another panic attack. Indeed, the health benefits of regular practice of any of these techniques extend well beyond the treatment of panic, as is documented by a growing body of empirical literature (e.g., Kiecolt-Glaser et al. 1985, 1986).

In those cases in which the therapeutic effects of relaxation are not felt as achievements of the self, there has often been an inability to make the transition from inductions performed by the therapist to a self-induced process. A long-term psychotherapy may be required in some individuals before the soothing activity of the therapist can be internalized and transformed into self-soothing. Among our patients, in cases in which such difficulties have arisen, the person has most often had a history of physical or sexual trauma; however, we have also known a significant number of patients whose apparently inborn hyperreactivity has been so disruptive to development that life has been inherently traumatic despite the absence of events more is typically linked with posttraumatic stress disorder (PTSD) because they are "outside the range of usual human experience" (American Psychiatric Association 1987, p. 247) or involve the threat of death or serious injury (American Psychiatric Association 1994).

Cognitive Restructuring

Cognitive processes are critical to the development and maintenance of panic disorder. Although just about anyone can have a panic attack under the right combination of circumstances, full-blown panic disorder involves not only physiological arousal but also the elaboration of characteristic—although often unarticulated—catastrophic assumptions, expectations, and beliefs, particularly the fear-of-fear process. These cognitive processes can be triggered by autonomic arousal, but they can also trigger, exacerbate, and sustain arousal. Treatment is most effective when both physiological and cognitive aspects receive systematic and coordinated attention.

We recommend that cognitive treatment of panic disorder be conducted with an approach that Hollon and Beck (1979) have referred to as "collaborative empiricism" (p. 180). Collaborative empiricism is a characteristic of the therapeutic alliance: Patient and therapist engage in a process of active collaboration that involves identifying problems, gathering data, formulating data-based hypotheses about the problems, and designing "experimental" interventions that test those hypotheses and generate more data for the refinement of subsequent interventions.

A critical goal of the cognitive component of treatment is modifying the relationship between physiological arousal and meaning-making. As previously mentioned, physical aspects of the panic state do not have to determine the meaning attributed to the experience of panic. When treatment alters how panic sufferers view the panic state, the state itself is dramatically altered.

Although there is no denying the physical discomfort of panic or other sensations of anxiety, less suffering results from the momentary sensations than from the sufferers' appraisals of the situation, the future, and themselves. The sensations are ones selected by nature to inform us that something dangerous is happening; in other words, they are *designed* to affect the meaning-making process. They do so in imperative terms that instill an urgent compulsion to seek and identify the source of danger and to take avoidant action. In the absence of any identifiable external threat, the cognitive course associated with panic disorder is to equate anxiety itself with danger. The state itself becomes something to be avoided, along with any phenomena that the mind comes to associate with the state in its search for meaning.

The resulting fear-of-fear syndrome tends to make the panic and associated anxiety states more impervious to reassuring feedback. The person in this state of mind cannot make the reassuring discovery that "there is nothing to be afraid of after all," because the state itself is considered dangerous. Panic no longer requires the validation of an external event. It has become self-validating and self-sustaining. With the panic state itself an object of fear, the panic-prone person's life becomes increasingly dominated by anxious apprehension of future attacks, a state of escalating chronic arousal that paradoxically makes future attacks more likely.

Conversely, replacing panic-validating cognitions with cognitive self-soothing mechanisms, such as those in the "AWARE strategy" presented in Table 3–1 (Beck and Emery 1985), can reduce not only the psychological suffering but also the intensity and duration of the panic state itself. Similarly, modifying the cognitive contents of a patient's anxious apprehension reduces not only the distress of the apprehension but also the chronic arousal and the probability of future attacks.

The first step in reorganizing the cognitive components of the panic state is to identify and articulate these components through self-monitoring. Once made available in this way, these cognitions can be brought under more conscious control and modified.

Self-monitoring is presented as a tool for data gathering and is easily introduced during relaxation training by asking the patient to keep a log of his or her relaxation practice sessions. Once the activity has been introduced in this positive context, monitoring of anxiety symptoms follows. At first, monitoring may consist of no

---

Table 3–1.   AWARE strategy

The key to switching out of an anxiety state is to accept it fully. Remaining in the present and accepting your anxiety will cause it to disappear. To deal successfully with your anxiety, you can use the five-step AWARE strategy. By using this strategy, you'll be able to accept the anxiety until it's no longer there.

1. **A**ccept the anxiety. Accepting means consenting to receive. Agree to receive your anxiety. Welcome it. Say "Hello" out loud or to yourself when it appears.* Decide to be with the experience. Don't fight it. By resisting, you're prolonging the unpleasantness of it. Instead, flow with it. Don't make it responsible for how you think, feel and act.

2. **W**atch your anxiety. Look at it without judgment—not good, not bad. Instead, rate it on a 0-to-8 scale and watch it go up and down. Be one with your observing self and watch the peaks and valleys of your anxiety. Be detached. Remember, you're not your anxiety. The more you can separate yourself from the experience, the more you can just watch it. Look at your thoughts, feelings and actions as if you're a friendly, but not overly concerned, bystander. Dissociate your basic self from the anxiety. In short, be in the anxiety state, but not of it.

3. **A**ct with the anxiety. Normalize the situation. Act as if you aren't anxious. Function with it. Slow down if you have to, but keep going. Breathe slowly and normally. If you run from the situation your anxiety will go down, but your fear will go up. If you stay, both your anxiety and your fear will go down.

4. **R**epeat the steps. Continue to 1) accept your anxiety, 2) watch it, and 3) act with it until it goes down to a comfortable level. And it will, if you continue to accept, watch, and act with it.

5. **E**xpect the best. What you fear the most rarely happens. Don't be surprised, however, the next time you have anxiety. Instead, surprise yourself with how you handle it. As long as you're alive, you will have some anxiety. Get rid of the magical belief that you have licked anxiety for good. By expecting the future anxiety, you're putting yourself in a good position to accept it when it comes again.

Note.   *Beck and Emery (1985) suggest saying "I'll gladly accept this." Some patients balk at the use of "gladly." They often prefer alternative phrasings such as, "I'm familiar with this. I've been through it before and I can handle it."

Source.   Adapted from Beck and Emery 1985, pp. 323–324.

more than a log of panic attacks with a numerical rating of their intensity. Later, more complex records may be kept. Specific self-monitoring strategies are described in the self-help books and therapist's guide previously mentioned, in David Burns's popular workbooks (1980, 1990), and in Beck and Emery's *Anxiety Disorders and Phobias: A Cognitive Perspective* (1985).

Self-monitoring possesses two distinctly useful aspects. One is the use the therapist and patient make of the resulting information. Information may be gathered, for instance, about the relative effectiveness of various relaxation techniques, or about the frequency of panic attacks and the specific thoughts that make the anxiety better or worse. This information is the overt or manifest function of self-monitoring, but a second, covert function is at least equally important: The process of self-monitoring transforms the very schemas it observes.

The simple act of rating the intensity of a panic attack (usually on some sort of subjective numerical scale) often changes a patient's relationship to his anxiety. The anxiety no longer is something that must be passively endured. In rating it, the patient is doing something, behaving in a way that produces a subtle but real shift from a passive to an active stance. Furthermore, to rate anxiety, the patient must step back from the experience enough to compare it with a range of past and possible future experiences. This process of active self-observation and evaluation of his own state tends to draw the patient into a stance that is both more detached and more masterful. The mere act of engaging in self-monitoring in this way empowers the patient while at the same time uncoupling cognition from physiology.

One problem therapists frequently encounter when a patient is invited to engage in more elaborate monitoring of thought processes is the patient's conviction that he has no thoughts when he is anxious: "It just comes out of the blue and then my mind goes blank" or "I wasn't thinking anything; it just happened" are common reports. Usually this is a sign not of an absence of cognitive activity, but rather of activity that has become automatic and unobserved. It is important to treat such denials respectfully but not to accept them without some questioning.

The following case vignette illustrates the type of discussion that takes place in the cognitive component of treatment:

Mr. A, a man in his late 20s, reported on his self-monitoring sheet that he had had no relevant thoughts prior to a recent panic attack that took place while he was visiting friends. "It was just an automatic reaction. I had had eight panic attacks there before, and I must have been conditioned or something, because as soon as I got in the apartment it just happened." The therapist agreed that the situation sounded like one in which conditioning might have been at work, but he suggested that they might still find it helpful to explore the experience further. He asked what it was like when Mr. A first arrived outside the apartment building—a point in the sequence in which Mr. A's arousal was presumably not so high as when he got inside, and consequently a point at which his cognitions might be more available to observation. Mr. A replied, "I was thinking to myself, 'Ha, I don't seem very relaxed.' I wondered if I should sit on the stoop and try to pull myself together. I decided that would be stupid. I pushed the buzzer and immediately felt trapped. I had this feeling of impending doom. I figured I had about 45 seconds max before they would expect me up there. I was feeling defeated and ashamed before I even got into the room."

Mr. A and his therapist were then able to examine the relationship between cognitive and affective aspects of the scene; for instance, how had it affected him to think in terms of "pulling himself together" instead of "relaxing"? How had this choice of words for the action he was considering contributed to his thought that using relaxation techniques would be "stupid"? How had the word *stupid,* directed against himself, heightened his anxiety? Did the rejection of the relaxation skills he had learned contribute to his feeling of helplessness and thus escalate his anxiety further? What alternative ways could he imagine talking to himself in such a situation, and how might they contribute to his feeling differently? Mr. A was then asked to think about his upcoming week and to plan an activity that would give him an opportunity to test out the effects of the alternative coping strategies they had just discussed.

Exposure/Desensitization

The essential role of exposure in the treatment of phobic anxiety was recognized even by Freud (1919/1946). He observed:

> Our technique grew up in the treatment of hysteria. . . . But the phobias have already made it necessary for us to go beyond our former limits. One can hardly ever master a phobia if one waits till the [patient] lets the analysis influence him to give it up. . . . Take the example of agoraphobia. . . . One succeeds only when one can induce [these patients] through the influence of the analysis . . . to go about alone and struggle with the anxiety while they make the attempt. (pp. 399–400)

Patients can rehearse all sorts of positive self-talk and coping strategies during their therapy sessions, only to find that their sense of security goes out the window once they are out in the world and experiencing their anxiety. The principle that underlies exposure is that one comes to terms with anxiety not by avoiding or eliminating it, but by reorganizing psychophysiological responses through practice in the state itself. A discussion of exposure and of the substantial empirical support for its value in the treatment of anxiety can be found in Barlow (1988), Craske and Barlow (1993), or Michelson and Marchione (1991), whereas Clarke and Jackson (1983) provide a detailed discussion of many technical issues that arise in the technique's clinical application.

Adaptive psychophysiological reorganization seems to occur most often under conditions in which arousal is great enough to access the relevant state-dependent learning, yet moderate enough to allow, with structure and support, the development of new schemas. In our clinic, we have most often found it practicable to establish such conditions through implementation of an exposure hierarchy. In this process, patient and therapist design a series of activities of gradually increasing difficulty. Beginning with an activity expected to elicit a meaningful, challenging, but manageable level of arousal, they gradually move through the series, practicing at each level of difficulty until a sense of mastery is achieved. Only then do they move on to the next task.

As Michelson and Marchione (1991) have reported, "Contemporary findings, culled from diverse studies, generally indicate that therapist-assisted, prolonged, graduated in vivo exposure appears most effective" (p. 100). In clinical practice, this has been the approach that I have usually found to work best as well. But approaches to exposure may vary on a number of dimensions—for example, the optimal intensity of elicited distress, the gradualness vs. rapidity of exposure, the medium of exposure (e.g., imagery, role playing, in vivo), the duration of exposure, and the degree of therapist involvement. As with relaxation, it has been my experience that different approaches work better for different patients. Just as with swimming, in which individuals vary in their preferences regarding water temperature or whether to enter gradually or jump right in, patients' preferences regarding exposure will vary. The therapist and patient collaborate to adjust the "heat" and rate of exposure to match the individual's needs and tolerance.

For each dimension of exposure, the therapist starts where the patient feels comfortable and moves toward a target behavior as success and readiness warrant. Frequently, for example, patients start with therapist-assisted exposure in imagery and progress to self-directed imagery. While continuing to do imagery work on their own, they may add therapist-assisted in vivo exposure. Whatever the approach, the ultimate goal is planned, self-directed in vivo exposure sustained until the patient has experienced some form of mastery in the distress state. Most often, this mastery will take the form of a reduction of arousal. In some situations, however, reducing anxiety is less important than decatastrophizing it by demonstrating that one can still function in its presence. With some patients, therefore, mastery consists of performing a targeted behavior *despite* experiencing arousal.

In clinical practice, patients often report that they have not performed a planned activity, but have nonetheless engaged in some other anxiety-arousing activity that arose by chance and would have been avoided in the past. I have known a few patients to progress successfully through an entire treatment program in this way, rarely following through on anything planned, yet gradually doing more and more. Generally, however, I find that planned exposure works best. There is a greater sense of mastery when one follows through on what one has planned. In confronting an anxiety-arousing experience, a planned encounter is inherently different from an unplanned one. In the planned case, the patient has actively *chosen* the experience, summoning the anxiety rather than being passively ambushed by it. The patient has chosen to take action, an action designed in collaboration with the therapist to provide a meaningful challenge while, as nearly as possible, ensuring success. Happenstance exposure is far less likely to strike this balance.

The patient's own physical sensations can play an important role in triggering panic. Increased heart rate, changes in breathing, altered muscle tension, or any of the other physiological sensations that occur during the panic experience may become conditioned stimuli capable of triggering either immediate, full-blown panic or heightened arousal and catastrophizing cognitions that eventually snowball into panic. Such symptom-triggering physical sensations are frequently referred to as *interoceptive cues*. The roles played by such cues are usually significant, although the patient is often unaware of their importance. Interoceptive cues should be screened for and treated through systematic exposure. Barlow and Craske (1994) describe a set of exercises—such as hyperventilating, spinning in a chair, or running in place—that can be administered in sequence to identify problematic sensations (see Table 3–2). These exercises can then be adapted as needed to provide graded, systematic exposure to the relevant cues.

To make the most of the exposure experience, structures should be provided to assist the patient in transporting new and adaptive schemas into the anxiety state. The opportunity to provide such assistance is part of what makes rehearsal in imagery or role playing such a valuable precursor to solo in vivo exposure. In therapist-assisted sessions, the therapist can perform a variety of functions, such as prompting the patient, eliciting relevant information about difficulties, and suggesting coping strategies. As the patient weans him- or herself from therapist support, intermediate supports such as flash cards, scripts, or tapes may be helpful. As

Table 3–2.   Assessment of interoceptive cues

Exercise	Physical sensations	Intensity of sensation (0–8)[a]	Maximum anxiety (0–8)	Similarity to natural panic (0–8)
Shake head from side to side (30 seconds)				
Place head between legs for 30 seconds and lift head				
Run on spot (60 seconds)[b]				
Step up and down stairs rapidly (60 seconds)[b]				
Hold breath (3 seconds)				
Spin in chair (60 seconds)				
Complete body muscle tension (60 seconds)				
Hyperventilate (60 seconds)				
Stare at spot for 2 minutes, then look away				
Breathe through a straw (60 seconds)				
Other:				

Note.   [a]0 = none, 8 = extreme. [b]These are alternatives; patient may do one or the other.
Source.   Adapted from Barlow DH, Craske MG: *Mastery of Your Anxiety and Panic II*. Albany, NY, Graywind Publications, 1994, p. 10–4.

much as is possible, the content of coping behavior should be elicited from the patient rather than fed to him or her. The therapist should always operate with an eye toward providing that minimum level of support that is yet sufficient to ensure success.

▌ Family Systems Considerations

In some cases it will be necessary to work with the family as well as with the individual. When a family member has panic disorder, the family system may organize itself around the disorder in a variety of ways. For instance, a husband may fear that if his wife with panic disorder ceases to be symptomatic, the marriage will break apart. Or a child who is the companion of a phobic parent may derive important self-esteem from that role. The inertia of the family system may work against the patient's recovery as the result of investments such as these, or out of habit, legitimate logistical difficulties, or simple lack of understanding of the principles behind treatment. If other family members refuse to make time or space for the patient to practice relaxation, make catastrophizing statements at the first sign of the patient's anxiety, or collude with the patient's avoidance, treatment will be difficult. A great deal can often be accomplished by providing the other family members with a relevant book to read or recruiting them as partners in the exposure process. When more complex investments in the status quo are present, family therapy may be indicated.

▌ Interaction Between Cognitive-Behavior Therapy and Pharmacotherapy: The Psychotherapist's Perspective

As I have noted, empirical evaluation of the interaction between cognitive-behavior therapy and pharmacotherapy has yielded mixed results. These findings become most comprehensible if we view them as a product of the clinical reality that combined treatment may be either helpful or unhelpful, depending on how it is done. It is useful to distinguish between treatments that are merely combined and those that we might term *coordinated* or *integrated*. In this section I examine some of the contributions pharmacotherapy and cognitive-behavior therapy can make to each other. I also look at some of the factors that must be considered for the combination to be an integrated and effective one. Whereas in Chapter 2 similar themes were addressed from the vantage point of the pharmacotherapist, here these issues are considered from the psychotherapist's viewpoint.

Especially at the beginning of psychotherapy, a significant number of patients are unable to participate in or to benefit from cognitive-behavioral treatment without the aid of medication. Some patients are so psychophysiologically disabled that they are initially unable to attend sessions either regularly or at all in an unmedicated state.

Mr. B, a 28-year-old man, was referred by his mother for cognitive-behavioral treatment of panic disorder with severe agoraphobia. Recently he had begun to have rage attacks as well, making him not only difficult but also dangerous to live with. After an episode that required police intervention, Mr. B made a series of appointments for psychotherapy, none of which he kept. As his mother described it, his attempts to leave the house would end with him on his hands and knees on the front walk, vomiting from anxiety. A prescription for a small amount of alprazolam was phoned in to a neighborhood pharmacy, and with the aid of that medication Mr. B was able to travel to the clinic and initiate pharmacotherapy and psychotherapy. During the early phase of treatment, alprazolam enabled him to travel to appointments, while the addition of imipramine eliminated his rage attacks and reduced the intensity of his panic attacks, making cognitive-behavioral treatment feasible. Mr. B responded well to psychoeducation. As his shame diminished and his catastrophizing cognitions gave way to greater tolerance of anxiety, his medication was reduced and his range of activity and mobility continued to expand.

Even when they are able to travel to therapy, some patients are unable to take in or use information as effectively without medication. Most frequently, the problem is that high levels of arousal interfere with the patient's capacity to attend to or comprehend the information being imparted. Less frequently, in cases of panic with obsessive-compulsive features, the patient may be able to listen to, understand, and recall information, but remain unreassured by it or unable to incorporate it into the schemas governing self-perception or symptomatic behavior.

> Mr. C, a 32-year-old man in good health, entered cognitive-behavior group therapy with a complaint of panic disorder with moderate agoraphobia. His initial panic episode took place while he was exerting himself unloading a truck. At the time, he thought he was having a heart attack. Whereas athletics and other forms of physical exertion had previously formed an important part of Mr. C's identity, he now developed the belief that any activity that led to a noticeable increase in heart rate was likely to cause a heart attack. He was able to hear and comprehend both his physician's reassurances and the psychoeducational information presented in group, and even said he believed the information "with part of my mind"; however, he was unable to *feel* reassured. Mr. C could not incorporate the information into his view of himself or into the beliefs that were activated when he noticed his heart rate increase.

In some cases of this type, we have noticed that treatment with an antipanic medication that is also appropriate for obsessive-compulsive disorder seems to reduce the fixity of obsessive beliefs and fears. It appears to us that the resulting increase in cognitive flexibility then allows new information to be taken in.

Just as pharmacotherapy may facilitate psychotherapy, cognitive-behavioral techniques such as psychoeducation are in many instances a necessary precursor to pharmacotherapy. A patient may resist medication for good, clear reasons. On the other hand, resistance may stem from mistaken beliefs, unfounded fears, or vague ideas or feelings that have not been thought through or articulated clearly. Pharmacotherapists typically make use of psychoeducation: information about side effects, mechanism of action, reversibility of effects, addictiveness, expectable benefits, and so forth are routinely covered, but such information cannot be imparted until a patient is able to make contact with the pharmacotherapist. The psychotherapist can frequently reduce a patient's resistance by providing information while also assisting the patient to articulate and think through values, concerns, and beliefs. Most clinicians are familiar with the delicacy of this process, in which the encouragement of self-examination and the challenging of misconceptions must be combined with respect for the patient's values and autonomy.

During the psychoeducational phase, proper treatment coordination dictates that both clinicians provide the same—or at least compatible—models of the disorder. Many pharmacotherapists will describe the problem as one of biochemical dysregulation requiring a chemical solution, frequently using the analogy to diabetes mellitus, a comparison from which the patient may infer that psychological interventions are of little relevance. On the other hand, some cognitive therapists may offer a model that views affects as entirely caused and controlled by cognition, implicitly suggesting that medication is an inferior or unnecessary option. A more integrative approach is suggested by Otto and his co-workers (1994):

> To give the patient a more balanced understanding, we recommend an integrated biological model that accepts biological differences in emotional reactivity, anxiety proneness, and anxiety histories predating panic disorder, while emphasizing self-perpetuating cycles of fear of anxiety and panic symptoms. Alternatively, if a disease conceptualization is to be presented, we recommend a balanced biopsychosocial model such as has been adopted with hypertension, a condition in which there is a biological loading that is modifiable by behavioral interventions. (p. 312)

Throughout the process of cognitive-behavioral treatment there may arise circumstances in which medication may facilitate or make possible a component of treatment. However, once medication has eased the acquisition of new skills, the problem of state-dependent learning arises. The patient's gains may be dependent on the medication and may cease to operate when the medication is discontinued. In our clinic, we have found this issue to be a problem only when medication has been maintained until after termination of the psychotherapy. In general, we have not found state-dependent learning to be a problem when a medication taper is coordinated with continued practice of the new skills within the context of ongoing cognitive-behavioral treatment. Otto and his co-workers (1994) report similar findings. Treatment should not be considered complete until any skills or enhanced capacities acquired while on medication have been consolidated during a medication-free period.

In some cases of integrated therapy, pharmacotherapy and cognitive-behavior therapy make each other possible.

Ms. D, a 45-year-old woman, requested treatment for panic disorder with severe agoraphobia. After a full year of canceled or missed appointments and extensive phone conversations with the cognitive-behavior therapist, she finally arrived for a series of appointments. Her coffee consumption of more than 20 cups per day was identified as an important contributor to her anxiety. Coffee was phased out and relaxation training was introduced. Ms. D reported, however, that she was unable to sit still for more than 2 or 3 minutes of relaxation practice before she would feel compelled to discontinue because of increasing tension on the left side of her head. At this point, pharmacotherapy was introduced. More than a month later, Ms. D., who was still unable to sit still for the relaxation practice, finally confessed that she had not been able to take the prescribed medication (fluoxetine) with any regularity because of a previously undisclosed pill phobia. Desensitization in imagery, combined with coaching on how to engage in positive self-talk, eventually enabled her to begin taking the pills regularly. Medication in turn enabled Ms. D to sit for full 20-minute relaxation sessions, first in the therapist's office, then with an audiotape, and finally on her own.

With respect to the relaxation component of treatment, I have encountered some individuals who have been able to engage in effective practice only after initiation of pharmacotherapy. Arousal will sometimes prevent people from following through with relaxation practice or even from deriving benefit when they do. For people who feel too anxious to practice relaxation, medication may reduce discomfort to a point at which they can begin to practice. The medication may then be phased out as the patient's internal self-soothing skills phase in; however, this process is not always a simple one. Some patients in our group program who have learned relaxation in this way have come to view the medication as essential for the effective use of their skills. Improper timing or lack of information about factors such as the sensations associated with withdrawal from a benzodiazepine may lead the patient to flee back to the shelter of the medication and to draw faulty conclusions about the efficacy of the psychological techniques.

For some patients, medication may be an appealing alternative to relaxation techniques for simple logistical reasons. Regular relaxation practice is usually the most time-consuming component in the cognitive-behavioral treatment of panic (although the exposure process can be quite time-consuming as well). With some patients, such as a single parent with small children, practical constraints can determine the timing and frequency of practice and strong motivation is required. For most of our patients, regular practice is the component of treatment most difficult to continue. Medication will sometimes be an effective alternative, but this choice should be carefully discussed with the patient.

When pharmacotherapy is combined with any aspect of cognitive-behavioral treatment, an important consideration is the pharmacological titration of distress. Here, again, thoughtful coordination of therapies is called for. Patients who are comfortable with pharmacotherapy will often choose to obtain as much initial relief from medication as possible, waiting until the tapering-off process to see if they really need to trouble themselves with cognitive-behavioral training. Even when they are interested in learning relaxation or other techniques, patients will often prefer to do so under conditions of pharmacologically minimized anxiety. However, when the goal is for the techniques to be available and useful under future states of distressing arousal, their chance of success is greater if they can learn and practice them in a more naturalistic state of distress. Pharmacotherapist, psychotherapist, and patient should work together to find the different medication levels that are right for the patient at successive stages of this process of learning and mastery.

Reduction of arousal will facilitate just about every aspect of cognitive-behavioral treatment. One of the foundations of negative meaning-making in panic disorder is categorical thinking, a process that leaves little or no room for shades of gray and rapidly converts even frustrations or setbacks into disasters. This tendency to view things in intense, all-or-nothing terms is the cognitive side of a psychophysiological condition whose physiology is characterized by states of arousal that are also rapidly escalating, intense, and lacking in the kind of transitional gradients that allow for the elaboration and consolidation of intermediate states.

Reduction of arousal, whether via relaxation or medication, may create the space for new states to emerge, but the character of these states will also largely depend on the cognitive schemas that provide their structure and content. It will be hard for an intermediate state to be sustained if habitual catastrophizing cognitions remain active. On the other hand, the catastrophizing cognitions may be accessible to modification only when they are tapped at significant yet manageable levels of arousal. When escalation of arousal is sufficiently slow, there is time to work with the cognitions.

In many patients, this *just right* level of arousal can be achieved through skillful or lucky cognitive-behavioral work. In others, however, it may be more easily achieved, or only achieved, with the help of medication. On the other hand, blunting of the arousal gradient via medication may have a less-than-optimal effect if the patient is not assisted to develop complementary cognitive processes.

Perhaps in some cases when there is no adjunctive cognitive-behavioral treatment, the therapeutic effect of medication may still be enhanced by the exposure that it facilitates. In particular, when termination of pharmacotherapy succeeds alone, without rapid relapse, this success may be at least partly due to a kind of de facto graded exposure to anxiety-related sensations that had occurred during the process of tapering off. However, the high rate of relapse associated with pharmacotherapy—particularly with high-potency benzodiazepines (Otto et al. 1992; see also Chapter 2)—illustrates how difficult it is for such a process to be successful without systematic support. The pharmacotherapist need not leave this support to chance. In the absence (for whatever reason) of formal cognitive-behavioral treatment, the pharmacotherapist can instruct the patient in the importance of taking an exposure-oriented approach to sources of anxiety. The stages of tapering can be made contingent upon mastery of mutually agreed-upon exposure tasks. The pharmacotherapist may also wish to recommend one of the good self-help books I have mentioned. In a recent study, Gould and colleagues (1993) found that for their sample of patients with panic disorder and mild agoraphobia, bibliotherapy using a self-help book was as effective as psychotherapy. To minimize relapse, treatment should be continued until coping strategies and exposure-oriented exercises have been maintained during a medication-free period.

When medication is used to facilitate behavioral change, one of the key issues to consider is how the method of change affects the patient's sense of ownership of the change process. Like Kramer (1993), I have known some patients to experience the effects of medication as freeing them to be their real selves for the first time. These patients report feeling full, immediate, and spontaneous ownership of the changes brought about by medication. Others, however, experience the use of medication as shameful, as a "crutch," as evidence of defectiveness, or as evidence of failure at psychotherapy or at life. Often, medicated patients can arrive at a sense of ownership of their transformation, and of pride in their achievement, if this goal is carefully attended to in the therapy. Negative feelings, inferences, and attributions should be sensitively clarified, understood, and respectfully questioned and discussed. Placing the pharmacological removal of distress within a context of comprehensive treatment also involving cognitive restructuring and systematic exposure is likely to enhance the patient's sense of ownership of the change process. With ownership come a variety of positive changes in self-experience that will further help to correct feelings of shame, failure, and defectiveness.

Many of the effects of cognitive-behavioral treatment of panic disorder can be enhanced or alternately achieved by medication. Medication ameliorates panic disorder by acting on its biochemical substrates to reduce chronic arousal, to diminish reactivity, and to blunt or block climactic extremes of self-escalating arousal processes. Furthermore, clinical experience suggests that medication, in some patients, will reduce compulsive or obsessive traits in a way that enhances flexibility of thought and behavior. These direct effects of medication tend to bring with them a whole network of adaptive sequelae. Reduced chronic arousal may bring with it decreased anxious apprehension and diminished propensity for catastrophizing and other negative cognitive patterns. Slowed and blunted reactivity offers new space for self-observation and cognitive mediation of one's reactions, and may decrease the physiological support for categorical thinking. Adaptive changes in behavior and in self-experience may spontaneously ripple throughout the patient's life.

Pharmacotherapy by itself, however, does not guarantee these psychologically adaptive results. Maladaptive behavioral and cognitive response patterns can become independent of the physiological and biochemical processes with which they first evolved. Negative appraisals, beliefs, values, expectations, and self-representations may persist in a mutually confirming cycle with avoidance, passivity, social skills deficits, and other maladaptive behaviors.

The resilience of negative representations can limit self-observation and the ownership of new capacities despite biologically effective medication. This resilience is illustrated by Donald

Klein's (1981) account of the failure of early research subjects to note the fact that imipramine had blocked their panic attacks. By employing self-monitoring, Socratic questioning, judicious mirroring, and other techniques of collaborative empiricism, a psychotherapist who is aware of the range and sensitive to the subtleties of the possible therapeutic effects of medication can greatly enhance the patient's own awareness of these effects. The psychotherapist is then in a position to assist the patient in maximizing the opportunities represented by the medication effects.

Once in the grasp of learned helplessness, patients who had repeatedly been jolted by panic every time they left the house will often have difficulty in discovering that the biochemical barriers to going out have been removed by medication. As Freud observed, this can only be learned by actually going out of the house—that is, by an exercise in exposure. And even if such patients do go out, catastrophic cognitions can so consume their attention and arouse their physiology that it may be hard to notice the difference without the systematic assistance of cognitive-behavioral interventions.

As I have noted, the fear-of-fear process plays a critical role in evolution from an initial panic attack to panic disorder. In a treatment that includes pharmacotherapy, it will be important for all involved to be mindful of the role played by fear of fear, and of how the medication is interacting with this aspect of the disorder. Medication may help a person avoid panic or other anxiety states. However, its doing so may no more enhance the person's capacity to cope with anxiety than the act of removing all the dogs from the environment of a person with a dog phobia would alter that person's capacity to cope with dogs. *What is important for enduring recovery is not that anxiety be avoided but that it be mastered.* Such mastery requires exposure, both to those situations that evoke anxiety and to the anxiety's interoceptive components. If medication is used to completely shelter the patient from the somatic aspects of anxiety, he or she can go through the motions of exposure without achieving any meaningful mastery. In this way, uncoordinated combined treatment may inadvertently foster avoidance of anxiety-related sensations and undermine the efficacy of cognitive-behavioral interventions. As Otto and his co-workers note (1994), it is particularly easy for medication to be used in the service of avoidance when it is taken prn (as needed). In a combined treatment, the pharmacotherapist should make a point of conferring with the psychotherapist regarding the patient's use of prn medications. Thoughtfully coordinated and integrated treatment may employ pharmacological titration of distress as a tool to maximize the effectiveness of the other interventions.

▌ Conclusions

Many of the advantages of pharmacotherapy are most useful at the beginning of treatment, when medication often works rapidly to reduce distress and restore adaptive functioning. Patients who need or wish to may then pursue other treatments with more de-layed onsets of action. Furthermore, medication can sometimes provide relief to persons who are unresponsive to—or unwilling or unable to engage in—other approaches or treatments. For some patients, pharmacotherapy can make participation in other thera-pies possible when it would not otherwise have been so. Pharma-cotherapy's disadvantages can be summarized as follows: Not everyone experiences a therapeutic benefit. Among those who do experience a therapeutic effect, some experience prohibitive side effects. Use of medication conflicts with some people's value sys-tems. Use is seen by some people as evidence of a weakness or defect in the self and hence becomes a source of narcissistic injury. The benefits of medication may be experienced as the product of external forces acting upon the self rather than as an integrated achievement of the self. Although it may alleviate physiologically distressing components of the panic state, and even modify how a person thinks while in treatment, medication itself does not neces-sarily alter the meaning attributed to the state, the person's psy-chological mechanisms for coping with it, or the cognitive or behavioral responses that the state will elicit when it recurs, espe-cially after medication is discontinued. Finally, and probably as a result of the foregoing factors, discontinuation of pharma-cotherapy for panic is associated with a high rate of relapse.

In contrast, the main disadvantages of a cognitive-behavioral approach to treating panic are the time it takes to work (usually a minimum of 12–14 weeks, and often considerably longer) and its requirement for a relatively large, persistent, and well-organized effort on a daily or near-daily basis over a period of weeks before yielding a substantial benefit. A significant portion of panic suffer-ers lack either the resources or the willingness to engage in this process, and many more are unable either to participate or to derive full benefit from the process without the support of medi-cation.

For those who are willing and able to participate in it, however, the main advantage of cognitive-behavioral treatment is that the results are experienced as a product of personal effort and as a manifestation of newly developed or discovered capacities of the self. Cognitive-behavioral treatment explicitly addresses issues of self-esteem and self-representation and the meaning-making pro-cess that surrounds the panic state, modifying how sufferers view both the panic state and themselves, as well as affecting how they will respond to subsequent episodes.

As I have emphasized in this chapter, in both research and clinical practice, it may be useful to make a conceptual distinction between *combining* treatment approaches and *integrating* them. When treatments are simply added on, for example, medication may actually work against long-term goals by facilitating undue avoidance of anxiety states or by excessively blocking the arousal necessary for effective exposure treatment. On the other hand, when treatments are coordinated and integrated, medication may promote the goals of cognitive-behavior therapy by titrating arousal while also sparing the patient unnecessary suffering.

Further scientific research is needed to confirm and clarify the possible differential advantages and pitfalls of pharmacotherapy versus psychotherapy and of combined versus integrated treat-ment approaches. It may be that some patients will respond best to single-modality treatment, whereas others will receive the most benefit from integrated treatments. In the meantime, clinical experience indicates that cognitive-behavior therapy and pharmacotherapy have clear potential to enhance each other's effectiveness in the treatment of panic disorder. When these approaches are combined, best results will probably be obtained when they are also integrated in a coordinated program implemented by a clinician or clinicians who understand and appreciate both treatment modalities.

▌ References

American Psychiatric Association: Diagnostic and Statistical Manual of Mental Disorders, 3rd Edition, Revised. Washington, DC, American Psychiatric Association, 1987

American Psychiatric Association: Diagnostic and Statistical Manual of Mental Disorders, 4th Edition. Washington, DC, American Psychiatric Association, 1994

Babior S, Goldman C: Overcoming Panic Attacks. Minneapolis, MN, Compcare Publishers, 1990

Barlow DH: Anxiety and Its Disorders: The Nature and Treatment of Anxiety and Panic. New York, Guilford, 1988

Barlow DH, Cerny JA: Psychological Treatment of Panic. New York, Guilford, 1988

Barlow DH, Craske MG: Therapist's Guide for Mastery of Your Anxiety and Panic. Albany, NY, Graywind Publications, 1990

Barlow DH, Craske MG: Mastery of Your Anxiety and Panic II. Albany, NY, Graywind Publications, 1994

Basoglu M: Pharmacological and behavioral treatment of panic disorder. Psychother Psychosom 58:57–59, 1992

Beck AT, Emery G: Anxiety Disorders and Phobias: A Cognitive Perspective. New York, Basic Books, 1985

Benson H: The Relaxation Response. New York, William Morrow, 1975

Bourne EJ: The Anxiety and Phobia Workbook. Oakland, CA, New Harbinger Publications, 1990

Brown DP, Fromm E: Hypnotherapy and Hypnoanalysis. Hillsdale, NJ, Lawrence Erlbaum, 1986

Burns DD: Feeling Good: The New Mood Therapy. New York, New American Library, 1980

Burns DD: The Feeling Good Handbook. New York, Plume Books, 1990

Clarke JC, Jackson JA: Hypnosis and Behavior Therapy: The Treatment of Anxiety and Phobias. New York, Springer, 1983

Craske MG, Barlow DH: Panic disorder and agoraphobia, in Clinical Handbook of Psychological Disorders, 2nd Edition. Edited by Barlow DH. New York, Guilford, 1993

Eaton WW, Kessler RC, Wittchen HU, et al: Panic and panic disorder in the United States. Am J Psychiatry 151:413–420, 1994

Freud S: Turnings in the ways of psychoanalytic therapy (1919), in Collected Papers, 4th Edition, Vol 2. Translated by Riviere J. London, Hogarth Press, 1946, pp 392–404

Gould RA, Clum GA, Shapiro D: The use of bibliotherapy in the treatment of panic: a preliminary investigation. Behav Ther 24:241–252, 1993

Hollon SD, Beck AT: Cognitive therapy of depression, in Cognitive-Behavioral Interventions: Theory, Research and Procedures. Edited by Kendall PC, Hollon SD. New York, Academic Press, 1979, pp 153–203

Kabat-Zinn J: Full Catastrophe Living. New York, Delacorte, 1990

Kiecolt-Glaser JK, Glaser R, Williger D, et al: Psychosocial enhancement of immunocompetence in a geriatric population. Health Psychol 4:25–41, 1985

Kiecolt-Glaser JK, Glaser R, Strain E, et al: Modulation of cellular immunity in medical students. J Behav Med 9:5–21, 1986

Klein DF: Anxiety reconceptualized, in Anxiety: New Research and Changing Concepts. Edited by Klein DF, Rabkin JG. New York, Raven, 1981, pp 238–263

Kramer PD: Listening to Prozac. New York, Viking, 1993

Luborsky L: The promise of new psychosocial treatments or the inevitability of nonsignificant differences: a poll of the experts. Psychotherapy and Rehabilitation Research Bulletin 2:6–8, 1993

Mavissakalian M: Agoraphobia, in Integrating Pharmacotherapy and Psychotherapy. Edited by Beitman BD, Klerman GL. Washington, DC, American Psychiatric Press, 1991, pp 165–181

Michelson LK, Marchione K: Behavioral, cognitive, and pharmacological treatments of panic disorder with agoraphobia: critique and synthesis. J Consult Clin Psychol 59:100–114, 1991

Otto MW, Pollack MH, Meltzer-Brody BS, et al: Cognitive-behavioral therapy for benzodiazepine discontinuation in panic disorder patients. Psychopharmacol Bull 28:123–130, 1992

Otto MW, Pollack MH, Sachs GS, et al: Discontinuation of benzodiazepine treatment: efficacy of cognitive-behavioral therapy for patients with panic disorder. Am J Psychiatry 150:1485–1490, 1993

Otto MW, Gould RA, Pollack MH: Cognitive-behavioral treatment of panic disorder: considerations for the treatment of patients over the long term. Psychiatric Annals 24:307–315, 1994

Shear MK: Panic disorder, in Integrating Pharmacotherapy and Psychotherapy. Edited by Beitman BD, Klerman GL. Washington, DC, American Psychiatric Press, 1991, pp 143–164

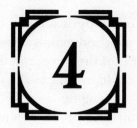

Survivors of Childhood Sexual
and Physical Abuse:
Psychodynamic Considerations
for Pharmacotherapy

Nancy Bridges, L.I.C.S.W.

In recent years, much psychiatric attention and study has been devoted to un-
derstanding the challenges and significant benefits of combining
psychotherapy and pharmacotherapy treatments for patients with
varying diagnostic conditions (Beitman 1981; Goldhamer 1983;
Gunderson 1986; Salzman and Bemporad 1990; Stone 1990;
Swenson and Wood 1990; Waldinger and Frank 1989a). The
sheer range and diversity of clinical target symptoms in patients
who have been sexually or physically abused would seem to require a multimodal treatment approach. Although combined
treatment is widely employed and may be valuable at varying
points in a psychotherapy with such patients, integrating psycho-

113

therapy with pharmacotherapy is a complex process. With trau-matized[1] patients, the psychodynamic meanings of medications, the idiosyncratic patterns of their use, and the intense and shifting transferences to care providers and to the drugs make combined treatment particularly challenging.

With this population, combined treatment works best when the pharmacotherapist allots the therapeutic time necessary to reach an understanding of the meaning of medications for each patient. For psychotherapists treating trauma survivors, it is useful to understand that medications may provide much-needed symp-tomatic relief from the acute and chronic symptoms of posttrau-matic stress disorder (PTSD).

Pharmacotherapy constitutes a potent, potentially valuable, and potentially disruptive intervention that will be inextricably colored by the dynamics of trauma. Combined treatment with this population requires both the psychotherapist and the medicating physician to be knowledgeable about the psychology of trauma. In this chapter I outline and discuss the psychodynamic features of combining psychotherapy with pharmacotherapy for survivors of childhood abuse. My aim is to educate both psychotherapists and psychopharmacologists regarding the symbolic meanings of medi-cation for this population and to provide a framework for under-standing the intense and varied transference reactions that affect other aspects of the treatment process. The medical management of PTSD is discussed in Chapter 5.

▊ Literature Review

It is well recognized that the process of introducing and managing medication evokes psychological issues that require psychody-namic attention to increase the likelihood of a favorable outcome (Beitman 1984; Salzman and Bemporad 1990). Studies specifically

---

[1] For the purposes of this chapter, *trauma* is defined as and limited to childhood physical and sexual abuse.

addressing the various psychological phenomena of medication management among survivors of childhood abuse or patients with a diagnosis of PTSD, however, are still unavailable. Recent research by Herman, Perry, and van der Kolk (van der Kolk et al. 1991) has demonstrated the correlations among childhood abuse history, PTSD, and the diagnosis of borderline personality disorder. Gunderson and Sabo (1993) have noted that borderline personality disorder is often shaped by trauma. Therefore, the existing literature (Brockman 1990; Stone 1990; Swenson and Wood 1990; Waldinger and Frank 1989a) discussing the use of medication and psychotherapy with borderline patients may indeed be applicable to trauma-surviving patients as well.

Havens (1968) examined the psychological reasons for misuse of medications among borderline and psychotic patients and found that patients may resist medication if their illness is serving an adaptive function. Waldinger and Frank (1989b), after studying transference and the vicissitudes of medication use by borderline patients, reported that shifts in the transference bear a relationship to the patient's misuse of medication and therefore must be monitored. Brockman (1990) found that medications may alter the patient's transference to the psychotherapist in both positive and negative ways. In addition, the pharmacological action of the drugs may be affected by the patient's feelings about the medication and its anticipated effects. Psychopharmacologists and other clinicians agree that the interaction between psychotherapy and psychotropic drugs is an area that merits further research and study (Goldhamer 1983; Salzman and Bemporad 1990). The dynamics—in particular, the transference phenomena—that operate in combined treatment, both with general psychiatric populations and with trauma survivors, have not been thoroughly examined.

▮ Psychodynamics of Trauma

A thorough grounding in the psychodynamics of trauma provides a conceptual foundation from which to understand the psycho-

logical meaning of combining pharmacotherapy and psychotherapy for traumatized individuals. Despite the vast array of
clinical symptoms and diagnostic conditions that may result
from repetitive, protracted interpersonal abuse, the damage
done to an individual's personality and psychosocial development and to his or her relationship to the human community is
in some ways predictable. Traumatic events irrevocably destroy
the individual's sense of invulnerability and distort and derail
personal development. As a result, issues of interpersonal control, autonomy, and initiative; wishes for restitution; feelings of
powerlessness; and anxieties about sadism and aggression become prominent and complicating features in all human interactions. The survivor's "emotional response to any person in a
position of authority has been deformed by the experience of
terror" (Herman 1992, p. 136). All human relationships are
tainted. In particular, those that involve an interpersonal power
differential produce a crisis of attachment as the survivor expects to be harmed or to do harm.

Herman (1992) defined and described the inevitable traumatic
transferences that develop in any treatment relationship in terms
of the roles of *indifferent bystander, perpetrator,* and *rescuer.* This char-
acterization of commonly occurring transference responses provides a valuable model for understanding the issues that arise both
within the survivor patient and between the survivor patient and
the therapist in a treatment relationship. The predictable reen-
actment of the traumatic experience—with its attendant terror,
rage, and wish for rescue—enters every relationship, and the patient's transferences shift among these different lenses. All relationships and interpersonal interactions involve these dynamics and a
very real sense of imminent danger. A relationship based on mutuality and respect, in which there is the expectation of being well
cared for and perhaps helped, is an unlikely transference possibility for survivors of childhood terror and abuse.

This model of the anxieties, fears, and wishes that survivors
experience in interpersonal relationships is relevant to treatment
relationships, because the psychodynamic features and transference responses that characterize and shape the trauma survivor's

personal relationships also affect the therapeutic interaction. Psychotherapists and pharmacotherapists can use their understanding of how chronic trauma distorts and contaminates the trauma survivor's relationships and sense of self to maintain their equilibrium and to endure the affective storms and confusing and difficult transference and countertransference responses encountered throughout the long, arduous process of treatment.

▌ Pharmacotherapy

Symbolic Meanings of Medications

Although the psychology and the neurophysiological responses and sequelae to traumatization have been well researched and extensively presented (Brown and Anderson 1991; Herman 1992; Janoff-Bulman 1985; Miller 1984; Sanford 1990; Titchener 1986; van der Kolk 1987; van der Kolk and Greenberg 1987; van der Kolk et al. 1991), traumatic experiences have not been shown to produce consistent Axis I or II disorders other than PTSD. Chronic traumatization has been demonstrated or implicated in the etiology of a wide range of psychiatric conditions, including mood disorders, anxiety disorders, chronic pain syndromes, personality disorders, somatic disorders, dissociative disorders, eating disorders, and addictions (Brown and Anderson 1991; Browne and Finkelhor 1986; Chu and Dill 1990; Herman et al. 1989). Each of these disorders may be treated with one or more pharmacological agents and some form of psychotherapy. In a treatment approach combining psychotherapy and pharmacotherapy, the patient and therapist pay close attention to the meanings associated with the decision to seek consultation and the ingesting of medications. The effects and side effects of the medication and the shifting relationships with the psychopharmacologist and the psychotherapist also require therapeutic attention.

Issues of Control and Intrusion

To the outside observer, it is obvious that chronically traumatized persons live with severe psychic, somatic, and existential pain. They reexperience the trauma in the form of flashbacks or intrusive and recurrent nightmares, employ self-mutilating and injurious behaviors as a means of tolerating and titrating psychic pain and maintaining self-continuity, and suffer a degree of anxiety, terror, rage, depression, and despair that others cannot imagine. At points in treatment, there may well be one or more pharmacological agents that could be helpful in ameliorating painful and compromising target syndromes such as depression or states of hyperarousal and severe anxiety. Yet it is common for survivors to wish and demand to endure these symptoms without any pharmacological intervention. When one has experienced physical and psychological pain at the hands of another person, particularly a trusted adult, one's object world and all relationships become colored with terror and the expectation of harm. Feelings of powerlessness and vulnerability must be avoided at almost any cost. For many survivors, the taking of medication feels like allowing their bodies and perhaps minds to once again be invaded and almost certainly violated. The idea of relinquishing personal control and inviting dependency on a medication exacerbates one's sense of interpersonal terror and is unthinkable. Issues of autonomy—of being and feeling in charge of one's self and interpersonal interactions—are reactivated. A steadfast reliance on the familiar, no matter how painful, is preferred to the unknown. Tolerating and facing unknown interpersonal and physical situations reevokes the traumatic history with its attendant affects of terror, rage, powerlessness, and shame. A sense of life-or-death urgency is projected upon the unknown or unfamiliar situation. Terr (1990, p. 37) described "fear of fear itself" as one of the by-products of psychic trauma. In her study of traumatized children, she found that formerly flexible children had "lost their tolerance for change." To allow oneself to take a risk—to forge into the unknown territory of whether a medication might be helpful—requires a modicum of trust both in the world and in others' intentions. Traumatic experiences leave indelible marks and shatter one's sense of basic trust in the world and faith in human beings.

Discussions and negotiations around psychopharmacological consultations and interventions work best when the therapist demonstrates respectful recognition of the issues of trust, intrusion, and control by keeping the patient well informed, educated, and included in all decision making. The careful building of psychological safety in the treatment relationship involves respecting the patient's feelings, autonomy, and decisions about whether to use medication to aid in recovery. Often, a functioning treatment alliance must be established before the notion of ingesting medications becomes tolerable. In the following case vignettes, two survivors describe their feelings of terror, intrusion, and shame about the prospect of taking medication.

> Ms. A, a 30-year-old woman, presented after her divorce with severe depressive symptoms, disorganizing anxiety, confusion about her sexual identity, and interpersonal relationships marked by emotional and physical abuse. After 6 years of psychotherapy focused on stabilizing her emotional and interpersonal life, developing self-care skills, separating from her family, receiving advanced education, and entering the professional world, she began to uncover horrible memories of father-daughter incest and brutal beatings as a young child. Flashbacks and night terrors left her sleep-deprived and filled with a panic level of anxiety and rage that compromised her capacity to work. When medication was suggested as a means of helping her with these symptoms, she responded, "Drugs? I'm not interested. It makes me angry that you even mention it. The idea of taking medication is like being raped. Having a foreign substance in my body, never! Who knows what it will really do. I'll manage on my own. I don't want anything."

Ms. A's vehement response illustrates the survivor's experience of taking medications as a retraumatizing assault on bodily integrity. Pills may be viewed as foreign, sexualized objects entering the survivor's body against her wishes.

Patients in many diagnostic categories refuse a trial of medication because they fear loss of control or consider medications "unnatural." The following case example illustrates the survivor's notion that even the illusion of loss of personal control will be physically or psychologically harmful or damaging.

> Mr. B, a 21-year-old, single man, was sexually abused between the ages of 5 and 8 by an older male friend of the family. He experienced severe, paralyzing depressions, dissociative symptoms, chronic sleep disorder with night terrors, and a constant state of hyperarousal. Although he clearly recognized that his depression and other symptoms were seriously interfering with his schoolwork and making it difficult to take care of himself, Mr. B chose not to pursue a psychopharmacological consultation, stating, "It's not a good idea for me. I can't tell my story to anyone else and besides, medications are not natural. Taking pills would make me feel smaller, weak, dependent. It won't be me. What if I became dependent upon drugs? No, I have enough problems and I need all of me that there is."

The survivor's transference to the notion of accepting and ingesting medications is likely to shift over the course of the treatment, sometimes in unexpected ways. Sensitively timed, serial discussions are indicated if the clinician believes pharmacotherapy might be useful or if the survivor is self-medicating troubling symptomatology. If the survivor is medicating him- or herself with nonprescription drugs or alcohol to manage symptoms, other problems in living usually result. Self-medicating with alcohol, other drugs of abuse, or prescription drugs may lead to physical or psychological addictions, unintended overdoses with attendant medical complications, and exacerbation of existing interpersonal difficulties. In such situations, the clinician should discuss the benefits and limitations of the survivor's self-help method and recommend a trial of a more traditional approach. The potential benefits and risks of this traditional approach—prescribed medications—need to be reviewed as well.

Issues of Hopelessness and Despair

In addition to the issues of control and intrusion, the notion of accepting medication for mutually agreed-upon symptoms and disorders has varied meanings for survivors. For some patients, the psychotherapist's suggestion that medications might be useful is experienced as a prognostic expression of the therapist's hopelessness about the survivor's pace or chances of recovery and may precipitate an exacerbation of feelings of despair. In some cases, such an interpretation may, in fact, accurately reflect the therapist's feelings. In a survey of 40 psychotherapists treating patients with borderline presonality disorder, Waldinger and Frank (1989a) found that therapists were most likely to prescribe medications when they felt pessimistic about a patient's capacity to use psychotherapy. The psychotherapist's pessimism about the success of treatment may represent the survivor's own sense of helplessness. The offering of medication may be heard as a signal that the therapist is frustrated or burned out, or that the inevitably intense feelings generated by the treatment cannot be held in the relationship. Psychodynamic treatment of patients with abuse histories involves creating a psychologically safe holding environment—that is, the treatment relationship becomes a container and a vehicle for the patient to reexperience, in manageable doses, important aspects of childhood relationships and associated feelings. The ubiquitous feelings of hopelessness, helplessness, and despair that infect the treatment relationship represent the survivor's efforts to express and master the affects contained in his or her original traumatic experiences. Therapists' understanding of these feelings both in themselves and in their patients is most useful. Honest, careful negotiations between therapist and survivor need to accompany any recommendation to try medications.

Despite documented clinical evidence (Nurcombe and Unutzer 1991; Sachs 1990), the existence of ritual or cult abuse remains a highly controversial issue. When a patient alleges such abuse, however, the very notion of taking psychotropic medications may be complicated by these real or imagined past traumas. It is common for perpetrators of cult and ritual abuse to drug their victims as they compel them to witness, experience, and participate in sexually abusive and violent rituals and acts. For these survivors, a psycho-pharmacological consultation may be even more terrorizing, be-cause taking medication is experienced as an exact reliving of a piece of their traumatic history, stimulating affective flooding and intrusive memories. Prescribing medication for survivors of cult or ritual abuse challenges their capacity to distinguish past experi-ences and feelings from symbols and reminders in the present. Exploring these issues must become a cooperative endeavor in the treatment relationship if medication is to prove useful.

Feelings of Optimism and Relief

For some, the invitation to discuss and accept medications to di-minish troubling symptoms is welcome. A consultation may be received as a comforting, caring act that imparts a positive tone to the treatment process. Survivors may feel that their history and their pain is being taken seriously. Someone sees them, hears their pain, and will attempt to provide the necessary tools for their re-covery. If the pharmacological agent indeed brings some sympto-matic relief, it may facilitate the possibility of addressing other issues in the treatment, may increase the patient's functioning in the world, and may add a measure of hopefulness to the recovery process. Waldinger and Frank (1989a) have suggested that a phar-macological intervention may stimulate and restore the therapist's feeling of optimism about the patient's recovery—a feeling that will be conveyed to the patient and perhaps build upon itself.

Survivors who look upon medications as a form of being res-cued from all the developmental deficits, delays, and sequelae of their traumatic history are bound to have a positive attitude toward the drugs, at least initially, and may search for just the right psy-chopharmacological agents. The survivor's idealization of the positive power of drugs to effect transforming changes is rooted in his or her earlier wish for an omnipotent, omniscient, protective other. Havens (1968) examined the use of medications among bor-derline and psychotic patients and suggested that patients may crave drugs as a means of satisfying deep, unconscious yearnings. These yearnings, if unaddressed, may lead to psychological or physical dependence on medications or to the inability to reduce or discontinue a medication that is no longer helpful or indicated. Despite disappointments regarding the effectiveness of the pre-scribed drugs, some survivors are interested and remain hopeful that drugs will be a significant part of their recovery. As one survi-vor stated, "I thought medication would help more. I'm angry I have to do it (recovery) all myself." Repeated disappointments may result in the survivor's coming to grips with his or her unre-alistic expectations about the drugs. The individual's deep grief and rage at how he or she has been harmed becomes mixed with a more realistic view of the multiple levels of his or her impairment and the painstaking yet steady process of recovery.

▌ Patients' Relationships to Drugs and Care Providers

The personality deficits produced by traumatic conditions correlate with the highly individualistic ways in which survivors use medica-tion. Chronic abuse in childhood severely affects the survivor's per-sonality and psychosocial development. Physical and sexual abuse in childhood also distorts and delays narcissistic development and results in particular personality difficulties. Crucial narcissistic devel-opmental processes—including developing a continuous and endur-ing sense of self, attaining the capacity to self-soothe and tolerate aloneness, experiencing others as benign and reliable, establishing mutuality and respect in relationships, feeling entitled to listen to one's inner experience and take appropriate action, and being able to take initiative in the world—have been severely derailed. Survi-vors misjudge how to apportion responsibility between self and oth-ers, oscillating between entitlement and inflated expectations and feeling undefined and undeserving. These unresolved personality development issues lay the foundation for the idiosyncratic patterns of medication use that therapists commonly see in survivors.

Medications as Vehicles for Symbolic Communications

Survivors with unstable or underdeveloped self-systems are likely to use medications as vehicles 1) for symbolic communications about shifts in their inner worlds and changes in the natures and tenors of external, transference relationships, and 2) for expression of various feeling states. The literature suggests that instability of object representations and relations is responsible for patients' changing transferences to the medications and may lead to impulsive misuse of prescribed drugs. Waldinger and Frank (1989b) defined and discussed the psychodynamic use of medication by borderline patients, emphasizing the importance of transference reactions to both the therapist and the medication. They recommended paying particular attention to the patient's transference responses, which mark the fluctuating shifts in the patient's view of him- or herself and the therapist.

Various transferential meanings may exist for the same patient. For example, in a psychotherapy in which the therapist had been idealized as the patient's "port in the storm," the introduction of medication caused the patient's transference to the therapist to shift toward a view of him as malevolent, intrusive, and controlling (Waldinger and Frank 1989b). By another patient, who saw her therapist as a supportive, comforting object, medication was viewed as a soothing presence. However, while this patient's therapist was away on vacation, the meaning of the medication shifted, becoming evidence of his wish to abandon her (Waldinger and Frank 1989b). Medications thus become an intense and valued object relationship that is subject to the same instabilities and transferences as is any relationship in the patient's life.

Because prescription drugs can be so intimately associated with the person of the therapist (Waldinger and Frank 1989b), the meaning of the drugs to the patient may fluctuate with the valence of the treatment relationship. Thus, medication may function as a powerful transitional object to the valued psychotherapist or psychopharmacologist, enabling the survivor to tolerate painful feelings, intrusive memories, separations, existential despair, or the pain of aloneness. Medications may also become a vehicle for the expression of rage, disappointment, or a rupture in the cooperative treatment relationship. It is not uncommon for patients disappointed with their therapists after a particularly difficult session to leave the office and ingest extra medication or choose not to take prescribed medication as a way of expressing their rage and disappointment. Sometimes patients honor their positive, affiliative feelings for their therapists by using over-the-counter medications to overdose rather than drugs received by prescription. The following case example illustrates how medications can be used as a vehicle to communicate positive feelings of attachment to the psychotherapist.

> Ms. C, a 30-year-old survivor of childhood abuse by her brother, presented with a lifelong history of severe depressive symptomatology, anorexia, and intermittent suicidal ideation with several serious attempts. After several years of stormy treatment with the same therapist, Ms. C felt more able to trust the therapist and to rely upon her for comfort and understanding. When hit by a devastating series of interpersonal losses, Ms. C once again became seriously suicidal. Sharing details of her suicidality and desperation with her therapist, Ms. C commented that when she decided to take her life and overdose on pills, she planned to use aspirin. Although she had in her possession both antidepressants and antianxiety medications, she would not use prescribed medications to kill herself because she wanted to protect her psychotherapist and pharmacotherapist. Despite the fact that she felt unable to go on living and that treatment may have failed her, Ms. C was clear in her intent to honor her feelings of high regard and caring for a treatment team who she believed had deeply cared for her.

Herman (1992) described the life-or-death urgency that survivors experience within relationships and their oscillation between intense attachment and terrified withdrawal. The same urgency and oscillation are seen in the survivor's relationship with medication. Survivors may alternate between eagerness to try medications and inability to tolerate the drugs in their bodies long enough to assess therapeutic effects. Many survivors possess an exquisite sensitivity to their bodies, and even slight shifts in somatic sensations may trigger flashbacks and be intolerable. Pharmacotherapy with such patients requires focusing on their somatic experiences and the effects those experiences produce on their mental status. Allowing the survivor to be in charge is essential.

The private manipulation of medications allows the survivor to move from a passive to an active role in an adaptive effort to titrate intolerable transferences and to manage overwhelming feelings without the shame and humiliation involved in interpersonal negotiations. Drugs can be controlled. Real objects and relationships feel unpredictable and uncontrollable, as do the attendant feelings. The following case example demonstrates a patient's idiosyncratic use of medication to control transference feelings.

> Mr. D, a 45-year-old survivor of sexual abuse by his stepfather and beatings by his mother, presented with a severe, atypical depression, an undiagnosed seizure disorder, and instability in his relationships and his professional functioning. After many years of consecutive, brief treatments, in the course of a psychotherapy with a therapist who he felt might be able to help him, Mr. D remembered and revealed his trauma history. As the treatment proceeded, he became troubled by the intensity of both the feelings he experienced in the treatment and those he had toward the therapist. When asked about his use of the prescribed medications, Mr. D revealed that he was altering the prescribed dosage because he felt it was "too much." In fact, each night he emptied out half or more of the antidepressant capsule until he felt it contained about the right amount, and then ingested that.
>
> A discussion followed of Mr. D's feelings in the treatment and therapeutic relationship that he experienced as "too much."

Cases of patients who hoard extra medications from their therapists and who experience these stockpiles as a source of great comfort or as a symbol of their enduring connection with the therapist are common and well documented in the literature (Brockman 1990; Havens 1986; Smith 1989; Waldinger and Frank 1989b). Medication can be viewed as a rescuer if psychic and interpersonal pain becomes unbearable, or as a useless bystander if the drugs do not ameliorate troubling symptoms, or as a perpetrator if the patient feels physically harmed by the drugs or the drugs cause uncomfortable side effects. The survivor who hoards a lethal amount of medications may be taking action as a perpetrator, relegating the therapist or psychopharmacologist to the position of helpless victim. It is worth discovering the survivor's exact transference to the medication and how that transference shifts.

Unorthodox Use of Medication

Deliberate deviation from prescribed dosages and schedules results when survivors use prescribed drugs to self-medicate painful internal states and block unwanted preconscious or conscious memories. Borderline patients and others with fragile and unstable self-systems use medications to alleviate internal states (Khantzian 1985; van der Kolk and Greenberg 1987; Waldinger and Frank 1989b). Clearly, survivors may be impulsive with medication and "misuse" prescribed drugs; suicide is always a real threat. However, the self-prescribed, patterned use of drugs becomes stereotypical for some survivors. The following case example illustrates such self-medication with prescribed drugs.

> Ms. E, a 25-year-old survivor of mother-daughter incest, entered psychotherapy with disabling, persistent somatic symptoms after a thorough medical workup detected no known physiological basis for her complaints. Having been sexually abused as a young child by her psychotic mother, Ms. E was distrustful of the psychiatric treatment that had not helped her mom. She was willing to take psychotropic medications to diminish her symptoms of anxiety and depression. Ms. E recounted her abuse history rather matter-of-factly and seemed not to understand the relationship between her trauma history

and her present difficulties. She resided with a female lover who represented her most significant relationship, although it was marked by intense, rapidly changing feelings and many crises. Ms. E received medical attention one weekend after having a stormy fight with her lover and ingesting additional medication that resulted in her feeling faint and unsteady on her feet. Upon exploration, Ms. E disclosed her characteristic pattern of medicating herself with prescription drugs after fights with her lover. A routine had developed of Ms. E's ingesting multiple doses at unprescribed intervals to deal with her rage and her fears of the relationship rupturing permanently.

The next case example shows how survivors may repetitively use medications to block preconscious or conscious memories with the associated flooding of intolerable affects.

Ms. F, a 38-year-old married mother, recovered horrific memories of sexual abuse by her father and images of being tied up and beaten bloody by him as her mother watched and pleaded with her husband to stop. She experienced severe dissociative episodes, protracted depressions with great despair about having a self or a life, and intermittent anorexia and self-mutilating behaviors. As a way of living with intolerable psychic pain¤and, I believe, of preventing herself from committing suicide¤Ms. F developed an elaborate protocol for ingesting multiple doses of prescribed medication and over-the-counter drugs when the memories, intense feelings, and dissociative episodes became unbearable. She conceptualized this behavior as giving herself a psychological "time-out"¤literally, as she would sleep for a few hours afterwards. Despite the willingness of the medicating psychopharmacologist to allow her much autonomy and flexibility in the use of the prescribed medications, Ms. F continued to prefer her personal mix of prescription and over-the-counter drugs to alleviate and manage her symptoms. The highly unusual nature of her medication use became an area for ongoing discussions about self-care, safety, and other ways to manage acute PTSD symptoms.

Ms. F's preference for her personal mix of medications graphically illustrates the survivor's constant conflict around issues of control and trust. Rather than surrender or completely submit to powerful objects—the care providers and the pills—she devised her own "prescription." Ms. F's overriding need to be in control and her firm belief that more bad things could happen to her led her to rely ultimately only upon herself.

Using prescription drugs in idiosyncratic ways, employing over-the-counter drugs, or turning to alcohol and street drugs are characteristic ways that survivors try to deal with the acute and chronic symptoms of traumatization (Khantzian 1985; van der Kolk and Greenberg 1987). Manipulation of prescribed drugs and the resulting over- or undermedication may be dangerous for survivors and frustrating for care providers. The care providers may only learn of the survivor's unusual medicating practices when there is an untoward effect or the pills run out. Issues of control, secrecy, and aggression are manifest in the survivor's breaking the rules for medication use. Often, the behavior is not reported to care providers because the survivor expects to be met with a controlling, sadistic response from them. The personal use of medication in this way is often seen as irresponsible or misunderstood as suicidal behavior. Although dangerous, however, these idiosyncratic schedules actually represent the survivor's best effort to manage feelings, memories, and dissociative states that otherwise would threaten his or her survival. Practices of this kind can be particularly dangerous if the survivor uses illicit drugs or alcohol, or has an eating disorder and poor nutritional and medical status. In such cases, the risk of a miscalculation and unintended serious harm increases significantly. A serious and respectful discussion, pointing out the risk of unintended self-harm and empowering the survivor by recommending other, less-dangerous methods of managing symptoms and internal states, is warranted. Medications may have to be discontinued or changed to ensure the patient's safety.

Treatment relationships provide a holding environment that allows the survivor as much control as she or he can safely manage. Although this stance of both empowering the survivor and discontinuing medication if safety is seriously endangered seems paradoxical, it is both therapeutic and indicated. The message to the survivor is that his or her safety comes first, and that the treatment team will be in charge until the survivor can competently manage him- or herself. Consultation—continual review of the current medications and of how they are being used—is useful. The high prevalence of substance abuse, self-mutilating behaviors, and suicide among survivors of chronic traumatization is well documented in the literature (Brown and Anderson 1991, Browne and Finkelhor 1986; Gelinas 1983; Herman et al. 1986; van der Kolk et al. 1991). Psychotherapists and psychopharmacologists vary in their willingness and capability to be flexible, relinquish control, and view consultations with the survivor as a joint endeavor. Such a process does involve some risk, and not all clinicians wish to participate in it. In a survey of 40 therapists, Waldinger and Frank (1989a) found that 68%–70% of therapists were unwilling to prescribe medications if the patient had a history of substance abuse (68%) or suicide attempts (70%). Consultations seen as a process of negotiation, with safety—not control—as the dictating parameter, work best.

Combined treatment with survivors requires a well-functioning treatment team with close coordination and communication between therapist and psychopharmacologist. Shifting and split alliances and intense and varied transferences among the treatment team members can mirror the survivor's experience. A treatment team that openly discusses and anticipates the replication among themselves of the affects experienced in the patient's traumatic past will reduce the incidence of reenactments of the survivor's history.

▌ Conclusions

Combining psychotherapy and pharmacotherapy in the treatment of survivors of chronic traumatization is a widely accepted practice. For such patients, the multiple and varied meanings of medications may range from a welcome relief, a sign of hopeless-ness, or a terrorizing intrusion. Issues of trust, control, intrusion, and negotiation of power remain salient themes surrounding all decisions about medications. Care providers' understanding and clarification of these issues is valuable.

Because of the personality deficits produced by chronic trau-matization, survivors may use medications in an unorthodox man-ner. Unorthodox use of medications may, at times, be risky and requires ongoing attention and negotiation. Ultimately, limits for safety may need to be set. Shifting traumatic transferences to the pills, the psychotherapist, and the psychopharmacologist are to be expected. The nature of the transference may inform treatment decisions.

Discussions and negotiations with survivors around medica-tion are likely to be successful if emphasis is placed on empower-ing and educating the patient. Control struggles can be avoided by focusing on safety concerns. The inevitably intense and shifting transference relationships among treatment team members re-quire careful attention. Open and frequent communication, mu-tual support and respect, and discussion of the shifting transferences increase the possibility of a favorable outcome.

▌ References

Beitman BD: Pharmacotherapy as an intervention during the stages of psychotherapy. Am J Psychother 35:206–214, 1981

Beitman BD: Introducing medications during psychotherapy, in Combining Psychotherapy and Drug Therapy in Clinical Prac-tice. Edited by Beitman BD, Klerman GL. New York, Spectrum, 1984, pp 65–87

Brockman R: Medication and transference in psychoanalytically oriented psychotherapy of the borderline patient. Psychiatr Clin North Am 13:287–295, 1990

Brown G, Anderson B: Psychiatric morbidity in adult inpatients with childhood histories of sexual and physical abuse. Am J Psychiatry 148:55–61, 1991

Browne A, Finkelhor D: Impact of child sexual abuse: a review of the research. Psychol Bull 99:66–77, 1986

Chu JA, Dill DL: Dissociative symptoms in relation to childhood physical and sexual abuse. Am J Psychiatry 147:887–892, 1990

Gelinas D: The persistent negative effects of incest. Psychiatry 46:312–332, 1983

Goldhamer P: Psychotherapy and pharmacotherapy: the challenge of integration. Can J Psychiatry 28:173–177, 1983

Gunderson J: Pharmacotherapy for patients with borderline personality disorder. Arch Gen Psychiatry 43:698–700, 1986

Gunderson J, Sabo A: The phenomenological and conceptual interface between borderline personality disorder and PTSD. Am J Psychiatry 150:19–27, 1993

Havens LL: Some difficulties in giving schizophrenic and borderline patients medication. Psychiatry 31:44–50, 1968

Herman JL: Trauma and Recovery. Basic Books, 1992

Herman JL, Perry JC, van der Kolk BA: Childhood trauma in borderline personality disorder. Am J Psychiatry 146:490–495, 1989

Herman JL, Russel EH, Trocki K: Long-term effects of incestuous abuse in childhood. Am J Psychiatry 143:1293–1296, 1986

Janoff-Bulman R: The aftermath of victimization: rebuilding shattered assumptions, in Trauma and Its Wake, Vol 1. Edited by Figley CR. New York, Brunner/Mazel, 1985, pp 15–35

Khantzian EJ: The self-medication hypothesis of addictive disorders: focus on heroin and cocaine dependence. Am J Psychiatry 142:1259–1264, 1985

Miller A: For Your Own Good. New York, Farrar, Straus & Giroux, 1984

Nurcombe B, Unutzer J: The ritual abuse of children: clinical features and diagnostic reasoning. J Am Acad Child Adolesc Psychiatry 30:272–276, 1991

Sachs RG: The role of sex and pregnancy in satanic cults. Pre- and Peri-Natal Psychology 5:105–113, 1990

Salzman C, Bemporad J: Clinical observations on the combined psychotherapeutic and psychopharmacologic treatment of the depressed patient. Paper presented at a psychopharmacology conference at The Cambridge Hospital, Cambridge, MA, January 6, 1990

Sanford LT: Strong at the Broken Places. New York, Random House, 1990

Smith J: Some dimensions of transference in combined treatment, in The Psychotherapist's Guide to Pharmacotherapy. Edited by Ellison JM. St. Louis, MO, Mosby/Year Book, 1989, pp 79–95

Stone MH: Treatment of borderline patients: a pragmatic approach. Psychiatr Clin North Am 13:265–285, 1990

Swenson CR, Wood MC: Issues involved in combining drugs with psychotherapy for the borderline inpatient. Psychiatr Clin North Am 15:297–306, 1990

Terr LC: Too Scared to Cry. New York, Basic Books, 1990

Titchener J: Post-traumatic decline: a consequence of unresolved destructive drives, in Trauma and Its Wake, Vol 2. Edited by Figley CR. New York, Brunner/Mazel, 1986, pp 5–19

van der Kolk BA: The psychological consequences of overwhelming life experiences, in Psychological Trauma. Edited by van der Kolk BA. Washington, DC, American Psychiatric Press, 1987, pp 1–30

van der Kolk BA, Greenberg M: The psychobiology of the trauma response: hyperarousal, constriction, and addiction to traumatic reexposure, in Psychological Trauma. Edited by van der Kolk BA. Washington, DC, American Psychiatric Press, 1987, pp 63–87

van der Kolk BA, Perry JC, Herman JL: Childhood origins of self-destructive behavior. Am J Psychiatry 148:1665–1671, 1991

Waldinger RJ, Frank AF: Clinicians' experiences in combining medication and psychotherapy in the treatment of borderline patients. Hosp Community Psychiatry 40:712–718, 1989a

Waldinger RJ, Frank AF: Transference and the vicissitudes of medication use by borderline patients. Psychiatry 52:416–427, 1989b

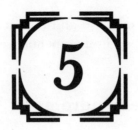

Posttraumatic Stress Disorder: A Collaborative and Integrative Approach to Pharmacotherapy

Pamela Reeves, M.D., and
James M. Ellison, M.D., M.P.H.

Posttraumatic stress disorder (PTSD), which has a lifetime prevalence of 8%–15% in the United States (Davidson et al. 1991b; Helzer et al. 1987), is one of the most widespread anxiety disorders. Growing awareness of the chronic, damaging effects of trauma (e.g., Herman 1992; Herman et al. 1986) has encouraged clinicians to seek effective treatment approaches. For many patients, supplementation of individual and group psychotherapy with symptom-targeted pharmacotherapy improves the course and outcome of treatment. In this chapter we review the syndromal definition of PTSD, several biological hypotheses regarding its nature, and the most credible studies of pharmacotherapy. To augment the discussion in Chapter 4, we then address the psychodynamics of a pharmacotherapy consultation and the incorporation of medications into an ongoing psychotherapeutic treatment.

■ The Syndrome of PTSD

To diagnose PTSD in accordance with DSM-IV (American Psychiatric Association 1994) criteria, the clinician must identify in the patient's life a traumatic event or series of events, the experience or witnessing of which led to intense fear, helplessness, or horror. The resulting symptoms fall into three distinct clusters: 1) persistent, intrusive *reexperiencing* of a traumatic event, for example, through recollections, flashbacks, nightmares, illusions, hallucinations, or reactivity upon exposure to reminders of the event; 2) persistent *avoidance* of stimuli associated with the trauma, as indicated, for example, by memory gaps, diminished interest, detachment, or numbing of responsiveness; and 3) persistent *hyperarousal,* as shown, for example, by sleep disturbances, irritability, concentration difficulty, hypervigilance, or an exaggerated startle response. Symptoms from one or more of these clusters must have been present for at least 1 month for the diagnosis of PTSD to be made, although symptom onset may have been delayed for years after the event(s). The disorder is termed *acute* when symptom duration is less than 3 months and *chronic* when duration has equalled or exceeded 3 months. A new diagnostic category in DSM-IV allows clinicians to assign a diagnosis of *acute stress disorder* to patients who, following traumatizing events, have experienced PTSD-like symptoms for less than 1 month (American Psychiatric Association 1994). The existence of a psychotic subtype of PTSD remains a matter of controversy. In one recent study (Kumar et al. 1994), psychotic symptoms in a group of PTSD patients appeared to be either primary or attributable to a mood disorder. Schizophrenia or substance abuse seemed unlikely to account for the symptoms.

Any of a large variety of stressful experiences can produce the syndrome of PTSD. Traumatizing events can be singular, such as an assault or natural disaster, or part of a chronic and repetitive pattern, such as childhood physical or sexual abuse (Terr 1991). PTSD can occur in a previously healthy individual, but also may develop in a person already affected by a psychiatric condition such as a phobic disorder, panic disorder, obsessive-compulsive disorder, a mood disorder, a personality disorder, or substance abuse. PTSD can facilitate the development of additional mental disorders, such as substance abuse, mood disorders, or (when physical trauma to the brain has occurred) organic mental disorders resulting in changes to mood, cognition, or personality.

▌ Pathophysiology of PTSD

A variety of hypotheses have been advanced to explain how traumatic experience might alter an individual's experience and behavior, leaving in its wake a psychiatric disorder. Early psychoanalysts proposed that trauma could reactivate unresolved conflicts from childhood, a view later extended by the concept that avoidant and intrusive PTSD symptoms could represent alternating attempts to cope through avoiding or attempting to master the effects of the experience. A hypothesis proposed by cognitive theorists is that PTSD symptoms represent the result of an attempt to process intolerable types or amounts of information, resulting in alternating states of avoidance and flooding (Kaplan and Sadock 1991; Kolb 1987).

Neurobiological theories of PTSD have been reviewed and evaluated by van der Kolk and Saporta (1991). These have included several hypothesized neurotransmitter or electrophysiological dysfunctions. All the suggested pathophysiological models focus on the brain's limbic system, an interconnected ring of structures intimately involved with drives, affects, and the expression of emotions.

A proposed abnormality in norepinephrine neurotransmission is consistent with the finding that PTSD subjects administered yohimbine, a potent releaser of norepinephrine from the locus coeruleus, experienced somatosensory flashbacks. A hypothesized role for serotonergic dysfunction has been inferred from findings of lowered serotonin levels in some violent individuals and from the observation that serotonin antagonists can produce increased aggression in response to stress. Animals subjected to an experimental traumatic stress become depleted of norepinephrine, serotonin, and dopamine. Endogenous opioid function, too, may be altered in PTSD. An electrophysiological model of PTSD's pathophysiology proposes that repeated stimulation of limbic circuits might lead eventually to abnormal and autonomous electrical activity in limbic structures through the process of *kindling*. According to this model, flashbacks or intrusive affects or memories are manifestations of abnormal electrophysiological activity (van der Kolk and Saporta 1991).

■ General Treatment Approaches and Studies of Pharmacotherapy

In the absence of a definitive treatment approach for PTSD, many different methods have been explored (Solomon et al. 1992; Vargas and Davidson 1993). Most available forms of psychotherapy have been applied, but few approaches have been subjected to systematic testing. Many psychotherapists currently favor cognitive-behavioral approaches. Desensitization, flooding, or implosion may alleviate PTSD's intrusive symptoms, although flooding can overwhelm some patients and lead to unwanted outcomes such as an increase in the level of depression or an exacerbation of substance abuse (Solomon et al. 1992). Cognitive therapy—for example, stress inoculation training (SIT; Foa et al. 1991)—has been used to restructure cognitive schemas that contribute to PTSD symptoms. In the one controlled study available, dynamic psychotherapy appeared to reduce avoidance symptoms, while hypnotherapy may have alleviated intrusive symptoms (Brom et al. 1989). Group and family approaches have been developed, too, that encourage patients to share and draw upon the stabilizing support of a network of others who have had similar experiences.

Pharmacotherapy has increasingly been recommended as an adjunct in the treatment of PTSD, but such use has been subjected to only a limited number of controlled research trials. Although numerous open trials and case reports help to explicate its role, only six published double-blind placebo-controlled studies are available at present. These addressed the effects of PTSD treatment with phenelzine, imipramine, amitriptyline, desipramine, alprazolam, and fluoxetine (Solomon et al. 1992; van der Kolk et al. 1994). The majority of these studies examined medication response among combat veterans rather than in patients whose disorders followed childhood physical or sexual abuse. Of two studies using phenelzine, one showed a positive response among combat veterans with PTSD treated for 8 weeks with that agent or imipramine in comparison with placebo. Phenelzine doses were in the range typically used to treat depression, 15–75 mg/day. Intrusive symptoms were more responsive to active medication than were avoidant ones. The imipramine comparison group, treated with 50–300 mg/day, showed a significant but less specific improvement (Frank et al. 1988). A briefer (4-week) comparison of phenelzine with placebo, reported by Shestatzky and colleagues (1988), failed to demonstrate a significant reduction of PTSD symptoms by phenelzine. Another placebo-controlled investigation, an 8-week trial of amitriptyline, found a decrease in subjects' symptoms of depression or anxiety and a suggestion of improvement in avoidant symptoms but no significant effect on intrusive symptoms. Doses ranged between 50 and 300 mg/day (Davidson et al. 1990). Similarly, a 4-week comparison of placebo with desipramine found improvement in depressive but not specifically in PTSD symptoms at doses ranging from 100 to 200 mg/day (Reist et al. 1989). Alprazolam, in comparison with placebo, appeared to have a nonspecific benefit for anxiety without addressing specific PTSD symptoms when examined in a 5-week controlled trial of doses ranging from 2.5 to 6 mg/day (Braun et al. 1990). A 5-week placebo-controlled comparison of fluoxetine with placebo documented a significant reduction in both depressive and numbing symptoms at an average dosage of 40 mg/day. Twelve of 33 subjects (26.4%) treated with fluoxetine but only 4 of 31 placebo-treated subjects (13.3%) discontinued the medication before completing the study interval. Although not statistically significant ($P = .171$), this trend suggests that side effects may have interfered with fluoxetine treatment compliance. The fluoxetine study, which included both combat veterans and noncombat trauma victims, also noted that patients who were "just beginning to confront the realities of their past trauma" obtained greater benefits from fluoxetine treatment than did patients who had been in treatment for a greater length of time (van der Kolk et al. 1994).

Among uncontrolled trials and case reports, additional support exists for the use of fluoxetine. In two studies, fluoxetine reduced avoidant symptoms of PTSD subjects (Davidson et al. 1991a; McDougle et al. 1991); in a population of emotionally volatile war veterans, fluoxetine was noted to increase subjects' ability to delay action (Shay 1992). Some patients may, on the other hand, experience an increase in hyperarousal symptoms when treated with fluoxetine or sertraline (Kline 1994). One group of investigators is attempting to predict which PTSD patients will respond well to fluoxetine treatment by examining a biological marker of serotonergic functioning, platelet paroxetine binding (Fichtner et al. 1994). The PTSD treatment roles of newer antidepressant agents appear promising and await further study.

Propranolol, a beta-adrenergic blocker, was found helpful in reducing hyperarousal and intrusive symptoms in two open studies of PTSD treatment (Famularo et al. 1988; Kolb et al. 1984) but was associated with relatively prominent physical side effects. Though a potentially useful medication, it has also been reported on occasion to induce dissociative symptoms (Finestone and Manly 1994). Another reducer of adrenergic neurotransmission, the alpha$_2$-blocking agent clonidine, has been suggested to reduce intrusive but not avoidant symptoms (Kolb et al. 1984) and may possibly be useful on an "as needed" basis in reducing self-mutilation (van der Kolk 1987).

Carbamazepine, perhaps working as an antikindling agent, has appeared to decrease intrusive and hyperarousal symptoms (Lipper et al. 1986) and to improve impulse control in a group of war veterans. Its range of side effects and the need for careful medical monitoring, including periodic blood tests, have perhaps relegated this drug to a less prominent treatment role than it deserves among PTSD patients. Lithium, too, despite a range of potentially unpleasant side effects and the need for serum-level monitoring, can be a useful medication for increasing impulse control (Kitchner and Greenstein 1985). Valproate, despite similar limitations, will probably be used with increasing frequency following the report of preliminary results in combat veterans that suggested beneficial effects of this mood regulator on PTSD hyperarousal symptoms (Fesler 1991).

Neuroleptics continue to be recommended as an adjunctive medication when psychotic symptoms such as hallucinations or delusions are present (Friedman 1988). When possible, neuroleptic treatment of PTSD should focus on the treatment of defined symptoms and be conceptualized as a short-term intervention. This approach will minimize the risk of neuroleptics' potential long-term adverse effects.

Some variations among study findings may be attributed to differences in methodology and patient populations. Reports have focused primarily on combat-related trauma sufferers and study durations have been brief. Much remains to be learned, therefore, about optimizing the response of PTSD symptoms to pharmacotherapy. Differential pharmacotherapy response between abuse and combat PTSD patients, synergistic effects of multimodal treatment approaches, the nature of PTSD-associated psychotic symptoms, and the effects of prolonged pharmacotherapy remain among the many issues yet to be subjected to controlled observation.

▌ Psychodynamic Aspects of PTSD Pharmacotherapy

Although medication choice may differ substantially, the stages of pharmacotherapy of trauma survivors with PTSD resemble those of individuals with other anxiety disorders (see Chapter 2, Table 2–1). Caregivers first must prepare and refer the patient, who is then assessed and engaged in treatment. The pharmacotherapist (who may or may not also be the psychotherapist) and the patient choose target symptoms for treatment, with awareness that the psychodynamic meanings of those symptoms may be intense, personal, and not immediately explicable. As symptom response to pharmacotherapy is monitored, therefore, the caregivers and patient work together not only to adjust the medication regimen but also to process the changes in functioning and experience brought about through treatment. As symptoms are altered, a powerful relearning process can take place, culminating in a patient's reacquaintance with him- or herself. Some patients choose to continue medications over a prolonged period, while others reach a temporary or permanent stage of medication discontinuation. At every stage, from preparation and referral through discontinuation, caregivers must keep in mind the particular obstacles that may block the PTSD patient's therapeutic progress.

Referral for Pharmacotherapy

Although many psychotherapists consider the syndromal definition of PTSD too limited to fully capture the psychodynamic complexity and individual variability of this disorder, such a definition can actually be very helpful in guiding the pharmacotherapy. The tripartite classification of symptoms into intrusive, avoidant, and hyperarousal categories facilitates the designation of target symptoms and the observation of medication effects. In determining whether a patient is an appropriate candidate for referral for pharmacotherapy consultation, the psychotherapist may find it useful to step back from a psychodynamic formulation to a more simple descriptive assessment of the patient's symptoms.

Enumerating prominent symptoms in this way can provide a rough index of how likely a patient will be to benefit from pharmacotherapy. Those troubled by prominent intrusive symptoms, for example, benefit with greater frequency. When hyperarousal symptoms are dominant, patients may experience a calming effect from drugs that reduce noradrenergic hyperfunction (e.g., beta-blockers, clonidine, carbamazepine). Although patients most troubled by avoidant symptoms seem currently the least likely to achieve further benefit by the addition of pharmacotherapy to their psychotherapy, a serotonin reuptake inhibitor may provide some benefit even in this realm. The best responses to pharmacotherapy are likely to be associated with better premorbid functioning, a shorter duration of illness, and a likelihood of good treatment compliance.

Patients with a pharmacologically treatable concurrent Axis I disorder such as panic disorder or a mood disorder are often excellent candidates for medication trials. By simply alleviating the symptoms of the comorbid disorder, medication may facilitate a patient's more active involvement in psychotherapy. When the concurrent disorder is substance abuse, attitudes toward medication and the potential for medication misuse must be considered with special care.

Pharmacotherapy Evaluation

The pharmacotherapy consultant approaches a PTSD patient with attention to target symptoms and concurrent disorders, albeit in the broader biopsychosocial context. During the initial visit, the consultant begins to obtain a medical history consisting of information regarding the most disturbing or prominent PTSD symptoms, concurrent psychiatric disorders, past psychiatric history and treatment, past and present medical disorders and their treatments, any history of substance abuse, the family's medical and psychiatric history, highlights of the patient's social and developmental history, and a mental status examination that includes a screening for neuropsychological dysfunction.

Although many patients prove able to supply all this information within one or two initial sessions, some PTSD patients require several or even many visits before feeling safe enough to provide sufficient information and to achieve an understanding of the risks and benefits of treatment. Both the pharmacotherapist and the

psychotherapist can provide support to the patient by acknowl-
edging how difficult it may be to undergo this consultation. Patients often find it easier to bear the anxiety of the interview when
they are reminded at the outset that they can interrupt or end the
evaluation at any point if they feel overwhelmed. Enhancing their
sense of control in this way may make it possible to accelerate the
evaluation process.

Choosing an appropriate consultant contributes to the likelihood of a successful intervention. Many psychotherapists rely on
a tested and trusted colleague for what may ultimately be a challenging collaboration. Regular communication, mutual respect,
and a shared treatment philosophy will promote a better outcome.
Such a consultation is often best undertaken within a team setting
that brings psychotherapist and pharmacotherapist into regular
contact for the purpose of discussing a shared patient's progress
and problems. When a regular team meeting is not feasible, it may
be adequate to agree to regular communication regarding significant treatment alterations, changing clinical status, or upcoming
events (e.g., a psychotherapist's vacation) that require awareness
of temporary changes in coverage.

Avoiding a "Retraumatizing" Consultation

PTSD patients, perhaps even more than patients with some other
types of disorders, may balk at the notion of taking medication.
Not unreasonably, an individual with chronic symptoms may con-
clude that interminable medication treatment will be necessary,
leading to an unending reliance upon medication for stability.
This fear may relate to apprehension over a perceived loss of control or of independence and autonomy associated with dependence on medication. The patient may feel reassured by
discussions of a limited treatment duration and explanations
about the nature of drug tolerance and dependence.

Some patients have developed, through hearsay or reading,
idiosyncratic associations to specific medications. Lithium, for example, may be feared as a "really serious medication" by some

patients, whereas others may prefer it because "it's a natural salt." To avoid unwittingly triggering a patient's unsuspected anxieties, a psychotherapist can gently explore the patient's attitudes about pharmacotherapy in general and any particular medications that the patient might fear in particular.

Many PTSD patients have already struggled to reveal their stories to a psychotherapist and have strong doubts about or objections to admitting yet another caregiver into their confidence. Some patients actually refuse an evaluation because they cannot bear to give a detailed history, and the consulting pharmacotherapist can help such a patient by clarifying what will and what will not be necessary to discuss. Although specific details about a trauma can be of much importance to psychotherapeutic work, they need not be discussed as thoroughly in a pharmacotherapy consultation as the resulting symptoms. At the time of the referral, the psychotherapist may, with the patient's permission, provide the pharmacotherapist with background history and treatment information in sufficient detail to relieve the patient of the need to "tell all" to another stranger.

Sometimes a patient will request that his or her psychotherapist be present for the pharmacotherapy evaluation. When all parties are comfortable with that plan, such participation can prove enormously helpful in gathering comprehensive information about the patient's level of functioning and response to psychotherapy. Before such a joint meeting takes place, issues such as location and payment need to be discussed and agreed upon.

The Pharmacotherapy Process

When successful, pharmacotherapy can enhance the treatment of PTSD patients by providing a calming and stabilizing adjunct to psychodynamic and/or behavioral psychotherapies. It can reduce the distressing, disabling symptoms that interfere with the patient's functioning in social, occupational, and even psychotherapeutic settings. Pharmacotherapy rarely eliminates PTSD symptoms altogether, but it can diminish their frequency and intensity to a degree that allows a patient to bear them more success-fully and to participate more fully in life activities and other treat-ments.

Trauma survivors are often sensitive to and wary of altered somatic sensations. A thorough discussion of the medication's po-tential side effects should therefore precede pharmacotherapy. Sometimes the side effects may mimic traumatic sensations or act as "triggers" for symptoms. Tricyclic antidepressants, often associ-ated with constipation, can be particularly distressing for a patient who has been sodomized. Serotonin reuptake inhibitors fre-quently cause nausea, which may trigger symptoms in patients who have been forced to have oral sex, or who had experienced nausea as a component of their PTSD symptoms. By determining which, if any, somatic symptoms the patient has experienced and explaining the possible side effects of the medication, the pharma-cotherapist can anticipate and perhaps prevent an adverse reac-tion of this type.

In addition to inquiring about somatic symptoms of PTSD, the pharmacotherapist needs to ask whether drugs were incorporated into the initial traumatic experience(s). It is not uncommon for patients to relate that drugs were given to them by perpetrators prior to sexual and/or physical abuse. The potential for a patient to experience the prescribing clinician as another "perpetrator" should be addressed, and the patient can be encouraged to bring up those transferential fears should they arise.

Patients with PTSD and a history of substance abuse often raise particular concerns regarding pharmacotherapy: the fears of jeopardizing sobriety or even of developing a new addiction. The pharmacotherapist can show sensitivity to these issues by avoid-ing, as far as possible, prescription of potentially addictive medi-cations and by educating patients about the dangers or safety of whatever agents are chosen. Many patients, for example, are sur-prised to learn that antidepressants do not typically produce a "high" and are not likely to lead to dependence. Clarification of the differences between use, abuse, and addiction is often helpful. If the patient is involved in a "12 Step" program and has a sponsor, it can be useful to invite the patient to bring his or her sponsor for a joint visit in order to strengthen the patient's support system through sharing of information.

PTSD symptoms are often exacerbated by the recovery of memories, reexposure to traumatic events, "anniversary reactions," or exposure to perpetrators or locations where traumatic events occurred. These "triggers" may occur at any point in the patient's recovery from trauma, and the degree of havoc they cause varies widely, depending on both internal and external factors. Such exacerbations can even be a signal of excessively upsetting exploration in psychotherapy, an experience that may be impossible to avoid completely but that should not occur on a regular basis. During such an exacerbation, which is usually self-limited, increased psychotherapy visits and behavioral interventions are frequently necessary and on occasion can be supported by temporary or more lasting changes in pharmacotherapy. When a patient requests acute relief through medication, it is important to clearly delineate the "target" symptoms to be treated. Some clinicians believe, although no published studies yet confirm this, that the serotonergic antidepressants strengthen patients' resistance to triggers by allowing them to more readily obtain objective distance from their intense emotions without going so far as to dissociate. Indeed, some patients who have experienced this benefit from pharmacotherapy find that their recall of traumatic events is actually enhanced, perhaps because of a reduced need for the self-protective effects of repression.

Medication Discontinuation

No generally accepted treatment guidelines yet exist that specify the optimal length of pharmacotherapy for PTSD. It may even be unrealistic to expect that patients with such a vast range of experiences, symptoms, dynamics, and life circumstances should be grouped together in such a formulaic manner. Treatment, therefore, is tailored to an individual's needs, taking into account factors such as response to treatment, intensity and character of residual symptoms, availability of supports, current state of psychotherapy, and the presence of psychosocial stressors.

Discontinuation, like initiation, is most successful when preceded by thorough discussion. Although the decision to stop a medication that has provided relief and support may be appropriate, at times this action is taken prematurely or without adequate exploration. Such a foreshortening of treatment can indicate a patient's impulsive wish to demonstrate greater independence or to withdraw from the perceived control of a care provider. It can represent a response to narcissistic injury inflicted unintentionally and perhaps unwittingly by the psychotherapist or pharmacotherapist. Alternatively, the patient's decision can represent a self-punishing act, an expression of hostility or anger turned inward. When the pharmacotherapist is surprised by a patient's sudden disappearance or cancellation, which often implies abrupt cessation of pharmacotherapy, the nature of the psychodynamics underlying this behavior should if possible be explored with the patient's psychotherapist. Addressing such behavior directly with the patient without involving the psychotherapist can actually worsen matters when the patient perceives the pharmacotherapist's recommendations as coercive. In many cases, discussion that includes all three parties to treatment allows determination of a mutually acceptable course of action.

A suggestion to discontinue medication that originates with the pharmacotherapist is sometimes perceived by the patient as an abandonment. Reassurance of continued availability can be very comforting in this circumstance. Some patients will accept and make excellent use of the offer to meet periodically after medication discontinuation for continued monitoring of clinical status.

When discontinuation has been agreed upon, the PTSD patient's medications should be tapered gradually in order to minimize distressing change and to diminish physiological withdrawal symptoms that can trigger PTSD symptoms. Eliciting the patient's input regarding a withdrawal timetable and listening empathically to fears of yielding up a source of protection can enhance the patient's security. Anticipating and discussing the possibility that a patient will experience symptom recurrence as a personal failure will increase the patient's likelihood of reconnecting with the pharmacotherapist should relapse occur. Both patient and psychotherapist can be asked to monitor postdiscontinuation symptoms, subjective distress, or any change in functioning. Any of these signs may indicate the need for resumption of pharmacotherapy.

■ Conclusions

Despite the terrible consequences of trauma and PTSD, there is room for guarded optimism in treatment. Working together, psychotherapist and pharmacotherapist can offer a patient valuable support by emphasizing that PTSD is treatable and that psychotherapy can be supported by appropriate use of medications. Treatment can proceed most effectively by allowing the patient as much control as can be appropriately delegated, by choosing and monitoring target symptoms, by thoroughly considering the potential therapeutic and adverse effects of medication, and by maintaining an open channel for communication among patient, psychotherapist, and pharmacotherapist. In this context, medication can provide an important adjunct to psychotherapy, enhancing a patient's ability to accelerate recovery and optimize function in social and occupational realms without inducing long-term dependence.

■ References

American Psychiatric Association: Diagnostic and Statistical Manual of Mental Disorders, 4th Edition. Washington, DC, American Psychiatric Association, 1994

Braun P, Greenberg D, Dasberg H, et al: Core symptoms of posttraumatic stress disorder unimproved by alprazolam treatment. J Clin Psychiatry 51:236–238, 1990

Brom D, Kleber RJ, Defares PB: Brief psychotherapy for posttraumatic stress disorders. J Consult Clin Psychol 57:607–612, 1989

Davidson JRT, Kudler H, Smith R, et al: Treatment of posttraumatic stress disorder with amitriptyline and placebo. Arch Gen Psychiatry 47:259–266, 1990

Davidson JRT, Roth S, Newman E: Fluoxetine in posttraumatic stress disorder. Journal of Traumatic Stress 4:419–423, 1991a

Davidson JRT, Hughes DL, Blazer DG, et al: Posttraumatic stress disorder in the community: an epidemiological study. Psychol Med 21:713–721, 1991b

Famularo R, Kinscherff R, Fenton T: Propranolol treatment for childhood posttraumatic stress disorder, acute type: a pilot study. Am J Dis Child 142:1244–1247, 1988

Fesler FA: Valproate in combat-related posttraumatic stress disorder. J Clin Psychiatry 52:361–364, 1991

Fichtner CG, Arora RC, O'Connor FL, et al: Platelet paroxetine binding and fluoxetine pharmacotherapy in posttraumatic stress disorder: preliminary observations on a possible predictor of clinical treatment response. Life Sci 54:39–44, 1994

Finestone DH, Manly DT: Dissociation precipitated by propranolol. Psychosomatics 35:83–87, 1994

Foa EB, Rothbaum BO, Riggs DS, et al: Treatment of posttraumatic stress disorder in rape victims: a comparison between cognitive-behavioral procedures and counseling. J Consult Clin Psychol 59:715–723, 1991

Frank JB, Kosten TR, Giller EL, et al: A randomized clinical trial of phenelzine and imipramine for posttraumatic stress disorder. Am J Psychiatry 145:1289–1291, 1988

Friedman MJ: Toward rational pharmacotherapy for posttraumatic stress disorder: an interim report. Am J Psychiatry 145:281–285, 1988

Helzer JE, Robins LN, McEvoy L: Posttraumatic stress disorder in the general population: findings from the Epidemiological Catchment Area survey. N Engl J Med 317:1630–1634, 1987

Herman JL: Trauma and Recovery. Basic Books, 1992

Herman JL, Russell EH, Trocki K: Long-term effects of incestuous abuse in childhood. Am J Psychiatry 143:1293–1296, 1986

Kaplan HI, Sadock BJ: Anxiety disorders, in Synopsis of Psychiatry: Behavior Sciences/Clinical Psychiatry. Baltimore, MD, Williams & Wilkins, 1991, pp 389–415

Kitchner I, Greenstein R: Low-dose lithium carbonate in the treatment of posttraumatic stress disorder: brief communication. Mil Med 150:378–381, 1985

Kline NA: Sertraline or fluoxetine in the treatment of PTSD: early responses positive and negative (NR246), in New Research Program and Abstracts: American Psychiatric Association, 150th Annual Meeting, Philadelphia, PA, May 21–26, 1994. Washington, DC, American Psychiatric Association, 1994, p 119

Kumar N, Kutcher GS, Mellman TA: Psychosis with PTSD (NR248), in New Research Program and Abstracts: American Psychiatric Association, 150th Annual Meeting, Philadelphia, PA, May 21–26, 1994. Washington, DC, American Psychiatric Association, 1994, p 120

Kolb LC: A neurological hypothesis explaining posttraumatic stress disorders. Am J Psychiatry 144:989–995, 1987

Kolb LC, Burris BC, Griffiths S: Propranolol and clonidir.e in the treatment of post-traumatic stress disorders of war, in Post-Traumatic Stress Disorder: Psychological and Biological Sequelae. Edited by van der Kolk BA. Washington, DC, American Psychiatric Press, 1984, pp 98–105

Lipper S, Davidson JRT, Grady TA, et al: Preliminary study of carbamazepine in post-traumatic stress disorder. Psychosomatics 27:849–854, 1986

McDougle CJ, Southwick SM, Charney DS, et al: An open trial of fluoxetine for posttraumatic stress disorder. J Clin Psychopharmacol 11:325–327, 1991

Reist C, Kauffmann CD, Haier RJ, et al: A controlled trial of desipramine in 18 men with post-traumatic stress disorder. Am J Psychiatry 146:513–516, 1989

Shay J: Fluoxetine reduces explosiveness and elevates mood of Vietnam combat vets with PTSD. Journal of Traumatic Stress 5:97–101, 1992

Shestatzky M, Greenberg D, Lerer B: A controlled trial of phenelzine in post-traumatic stress disorder. Psychiatry Res 24:149–
155, 1988

Solomon SD, Gerrity ET, Muff AM: Efficacy of treatments for
post-traumatic stress disorder. JAMA 268:633–638, 1992

Terr LC: Childhood traumas: an outline and overview. Am J Psychiatry 148:10–20, 1991

van der Kolk BA: The drug treatment of post-traumatic stress disorder. J Affect Disord 13:203–213, 1987

van der Kolk BA, Saporta J: The biological response to psychic
trauma: mechanisms and treatment of intrusion and numbing.
Anxiety Research 4:199–212, 1991

van der Kolk BA, Dreyfuss D, Micaels M, et al: Fluoxetine in posttraumatic stress disorder. J Clin Psychiatry 55:517–522, 1994

Vargas MA, Davidson J: Post-traumatic stress disorder. Psychiatr
Clin North Am 4:737–748, 1993

Obsessive-Compulsive Disorder: Integration of Cognitive-Behavior Therapy With Pharmacotherapy

Allen Sherman, Ph.D.,
James M. Ellison, M.D., M.P.H., and
Satori Iwamoto, M.D., Ph.D.

During the past decade, a wealth of new information about obsessive-compulsive disorder (OCD) and its treatment has led to fundamental shifts in our understanding of the disorder. As with other disorders that are veiled by sufferers' embarrassment, even the actual prevalence of OCD had been uncertain. As scientific and media attention have begun to lift the shroud of secrecy, however, it has become clear that OCD is much more common than was previously believed; indeed, with a lifetime prevalence estimated at 2% (Karno et al. 1988; Robins et al. 1984), OCD is roughly as common as panic disorder.

Broader awareness of OCD has been complemented by the development of effective new treatment approaches. What was once regarded as an exceptionally treatment-resistant condition is now understood to be highly amenable to appropriate behavioral and pharmacological interventions. In conjunction with ongoing work in biochemistry, genetics, and neuroimaging technology, the new epidemiological and treatment findings have ushered in an era of greater hope for OCD patients while also prompting a surge of interest among researchers and clinicians.

▌ Diagnostic Considerations and Comorbidity

The principal diagnostic features of OCD, drawn from the fourth edition of the *Diagnostic and Statistical Manual of Mental Disorders* (DSM-IV; American Psychiatric Association 1994), are listed in Table 6–1. *Obsessions* consist of recurrent, intrusive thoughts, impulses, or images. *Compulsions* are purposive, repetitive behaviors or thoughts intended to neutralize the obsessive concerns. These symptoms cause significant distress or impairment, and, at least at some point during the disorder, they are recognized by the bearer as disproportionate and unreasonable. Common obsessions include fear of contamination by dirt or germs, concern that a disaster will occur because a task has not been thoroughly completed, and fears of acting on embarrassing sexual impulses or dangerous aggressive urges. Common compulsions include cleaning, checking, and counting. OCD patients may try to counter obsessive fears by employing hidden cognitive rituals, such as magic phrases, repeated prayers, or "good" numbers, as well as overt behavioral rituals such as washing or checking. These important mental rituals, newly included in the DSM-IV criteria, are often unassessed and therefore undetected by clinicians. In addition to active rituals or cognitive compulsions, OCD patients may engage in an extensive range of avoidance behavior, designed to distance themselves from distressing obsessional cues and to circumvent the need for exhausting ritu-

---

Table 6–1.   DSM-IV diagnostic criteria for obsessive-compulsive disorder

---

A.   Either obsessions or compulsions:

Obsessions as defined by (1), (2), (3), and (4):

    (1)   recurrent and persistent thoughts, impulses, or images that are experienced, at some time during the disturbance, as intrusive and inappropriate and that cause marked anxiety or distress

    (2)   the thoughts, impulses, or images are not simply excessive worries about real-life problems

    (3)   the person attempts to ignore or suppress such thoughts, impulses, or images, or to neutralize them with some other thought or action

    (4)   the person recognizes that the obsessional thoughts, impulses, or images are a product of his or her own mind (not imposed from without as in thought insertion)

Compulsions as defined by (1) and (2):

    (1)   repetitive behaviors (e.g., hand washing, ordering, checking) or mental acts (e.g., praying, counting, repeating words silently) that the person feels driven to perform in response to an obsession, or according to rules that must be applied rigidly

    (2)   the behaviors or mental acts are aimed at preventing or reducing distress or preventing some dreaded event or situation; however, these behaviors or mental acts either are not connected in a realistic way with what they are designed to neutralize or prevent or are clearly excessive

B.   At some point during the course of the disorder, the person has recognized that the obsessions or compulsions are excessive or unreasonable.   **Note:** This does not apply to children.

C.   The obsessions or compulsions cause marked distress, are time consuming (take more than 1 hour a day), or significantly interfere with the person's normal routine, occupational (or academic) functioning, or usual social activities or relationships.

D.   If another Axis I disorder is present, the content of the obsessions or compulsions is not restricted to it (e.g., preoccupation with food in the presence of an eating disorder; hair pulling in the presence of trichotillomania; concern with appearance in the presence of body dysmorphic disorder; preoccupation with drugs in the presence of a substance use disorder; preoccupation with having a serious illness in the presence of hypochondriasis; preoccupation with sexual urges or fantasies in the presence of a paraphilia; or guilty ruminations in the presence of major depressive disorder).

(continued)

Table 6–1.	DSM-IV diagnostic criteria for obsessive-compulsive disorder (*continued*)

E. The disturbance is not due to the direct physiological effects of a substance (e.g., a drug of abuse, a medication) or a general medical condition.

Specify if:

With Poor Insight: if, for most of the time during the current episode, the person does not recognize that the obsessions and compulsions are excessive or unreasonable

Source.   Reprinted from American Psychiatric Association: *Diagnostic and Statistical Manual of Mental Disorders, 4th Edition.* Washington, DC, American Psychiatric Association, 1994, pp. 422–423. Used with permission.

als. For some patients, passive avoidance is a greater source of impairment than active ritualizing.

OCD typically begins in adolescence or early adulthood, but onset can also occur during early childhood. Roughly two-thirds of those with the disorder have developed symptoms by age 25 (Rasmussen and Eisen 1990). Most OCD patients experience a chronic waxing and waning course (Rasmussen and Eisen 1991).

Depending on the predominant symptoms, OCD is often categorized into different subtypes, such as "washing," "checking," "pure obsessions," or "primary obsessional slowness." Different authors have proposed varying classifications (e.g., Goodman et al. 1989b; Zohar and Pato 1991). Although subtyping provides some useful clinical information, the relevance of such categorizations to etiology, treatment planning, or prognosis remains uncertain (Rasmussen and Eisen 1991; Steketee 1993). Most patients struggle with multiple rather than single OCD symptoms (e.g., both checking and cleaning). Furthermore, the predominant symptom often shifts over time, so that an individual troubled by compulsive cleaning as a youngster may present with debilitating checking compulsions as an adult (Zohar-Kadouch et al. 1989). Finally, in families with multiple OCD sufferers, sometimes each member manifests a different subtype (Rasmussen and Eisen 1991). Despite such arguments in support of the homogeneity of this disorder, it is clear that certain patient characteristics and symptom clusters predict differential treatment responsiveness. Among those patients who are likely to require modifications in treatment are those who fail to recognize that their symptoms are "excessive" (designated "with poor insight" in DSM-IV), those struggling with obsessional slowness, and those with obsessions but no rituals.

Comorbid psychiatric disorders may also influence treatment outcome. The majority of OCD patients present with coexisting psychiatric conditions (Rasmussen and Tsuang 1986). Major depression is the most frequent comorbid disorder; it is found to be present at assessment in nearly one-third of OCD patients, while two-thirds of OCD patients report a lifetime history of major depression (Karno et al. 1988; Rasmussen and Eisen 1989). Concurrent anxiety disorders are also common, with simple phobia, social phobia, and panic disorder of particular note (Barlow et al. 1986; Karno et al. 1988; Rasmussen and Eisen 1989). Coexisting personality disorders have been diagnosed in roughly one-half of OCD patients. Most frequently, these include avoidant, dependent, histrionic, or schizotypal personality disorders (Baer et al. 1990; Steketee 1990). Obsessive-compulsive personality disorder (OCPD) is often confused with OCD, but in fact occurs in only a minority of OCD patients—an estimated 25% (Baer et al. 1990). A principal distinction between these two disorders is that OCD patients, unlike OCPD patients, typically experience their symptoms as ego-alien and intrusive.

In recent years, interesting similarities in symptomatology, family history, and treatment response have been noted between OCD and a number of other clinical disorders (Hollander 1991; Jenike 1990b). In particular, a group of disorders appear to share the capacity to respond to serotonin reuptake–inhibiting medications. These observations have led to the concept of a hypothetical OCD-related illness spectrum that includes trichotillomania (compulsive hair pulling), body dysmorphic disorder (obsessive concern that one's physical appearance is deformed), bowel obsessions, hypochondriasis, Tourette's syndrome, depersonalization disorder, anorexia nervosa, and bulimia. The hypothetical "OCD spectrum" is currently a subject of intensive debate.

▌ Emergence of Effective Treatments

Until the late 1960s, the quest for effective treatments for OCD had been a disappointing enterprise. Although OCD symptoms easily lend themselves to classical psychodynamic formulations and contributed to early theory-building in psychoanalysis, psychodynamic therapy had been of limited help in ameliorating actual obsessions and compulsions. Standard behavioral interventions such as relaxation training or systematic desensitization, widely used with other anxiety disorders, had likewise yielded disappointing results. Traditional anxiolytic or antidepressant medications, for the most part, had provided limited benefit for OCD patients. Few gains and significant risks were associated with the protracted neuroleptic or convulsive therapies often employed in the effort to ameliorate OCD symptoms. This bleak treatment picture began to shift as new developments in behavior therapy, especially exposure therapy, paralleled advances in pharmacotherapy—specifically, the introduction of potent serotonin reuptake inhibitors.

The introduction of selective serotonin reuptake inhibitors (SSRIs), beginning with clomipramine and followed by other more purely selective compounds, profoundly affected the pharmacotherapy of OCD. Multiple placebo-controlled outcome studies of clomipramine (Insel et al. 1983; Jaskari 1980; Kasvikis and Marks 1988, Marks et al. 1980, 1988; Mavissakalian et al. 1985; Montgomery 1980; Thorén et al. 1980), including a large multicenter Ciba-Geigy–sponsored study (Clomipramine Collaborative Study Group 1991), have demonstrated the efficacy of this medication in treating OCD. Controlled trials have also supported the effectiveness of fluoxetine (Pigott et al. 1990; Turner et al. 1985), sertraline (Chouinard et al. 1990), and fluvoxamine (Goodman et al. 1989a, 1990b; Jenike et al. 1990; Perse et al. 1987). Although the response to pharmacotherapy is often only partial, the intensity of obsessions and compulsions is usually considerably reduced, resulting in dramatic differences in the lives of those who have suffered incapacitating symptoms.

Notwithstanding its benefits, pharmacotherapy's limits are evident. Some patients refuse medications altogether, irrespective of their efficacy. Others experience discomfort from medication side effects. Among medicated patients, a disconcertingly large number do not respond significantly. As many as 40%–60% of patients fail to benefit from initial treatment with an SSRI (Goodman et al. 1992), and although some respond more favorably to alternative SSRIs, monoamine oxidase inhibitors (MAOIs), or the addition of augmenting agents, a considerable number remain unhelped. Furthermore, for those who do respond, there are few data available concerning the persistence of pharmacotherapy's effects on OCD symptoms. Finally, relapse rates following discontinuation of pharmacotherapy are notoriously high. In one study, for example, close to 90% of OCD subjects successfully treated with clomipramine relapsed within 7 weeks of its discontinuation (Pato et al. 1988). The findings of these studies suggest the troubling possibility that patients relying solely on pharmacotherapy may require this treatment for an extended, perhaps lifelong course. Each of these concerns highlights the value of developing and implementing effective nonpharmacological treatments. Behavior therapy, although not without its own set of limitations, has been a useful adjunct or alternative.

▌ Overview of Behavioral
Treatment of OCD

The successful behavioral treatment of OCD began with the pioneering work of Victor Meyer (1966; Meyer and Levy 1973; Meyer et al. 1974) in Britain. In an inpatient setting, Meyer focused on blocking patients' rituals while systematically exposing them to the situations that elicited obsessional fears and urges to ritualize. "Apotrepic therapy," as he termed it, produced impressive results in initial trials with 15 patients. Most of these individuals maintained their gains throughout follow-up periods of 5–6 years. Meyer's work was quickly replicated and extended by investigators at the Maudsley Hospital (e.g., Rachman et al. 1971), and then by research teams in Holland (e.g., Emmelkamp and van Kraanen 1977), Greece (e.g., Boulougouris and Bassiakos 1973), and the United States (e.g., Foa and Goldstein 1978). The results of multiple controlled investigations have consistently shown improvement in 60%–90% of patients who complete behavioral treatment. Gains are typically maintained throughout 4–5 years of follow-up, sometimes with additional sessions (for reviews, see Abel 1993; Baer and Minichiello 1990; Foa et al. 1985; Marks 1981; Rachman and Hodgson 1980; Steketee and Tynes 1991). Although early research was done primarily in inpatient settings, outpatient OCD treatment has subsequently become the norm.

Behavioral treatment focuses on teaching self-management skills. Patients are invited to form a collaborative relationship with their therapist as a "co-investigator" of their OCD, thereby becoming active agents in their own treatment. Home training is an important part of the process. As they develop skills to monitor and alter their symptoms, patients generally experience a heightened sense of mastery, gains in self-confidence, and improved mood. Behavior therapy, however, can be a stressful, anxiety-provoking experience that requires a considerable investment of time and energy. Also, as with pharmacotherapy, symptoms are rarely completely eliminated, nor can every patient be expected to respond to behavior therapy.

The heart of behavioral treatment consists of *exposure therapy* with *response prevention*. Exposure therapy involves a systematic confrontation of the patient with the cues that elicit obsessions or rituals. A patient with cleaning compulsions, for example, might practice exposing herself to clothes she perceives as contaminated by dirt and germs. Response prevention indicates blocking of ritualizing or avoidant behavior. The patient with cleaning compulsions, for example, would not be permitted to wash her hands or shower after touching contaminated objects. By remaining fully in contact with the upsetting situation, without ritualizing or avoiding it, the patient undergoes a relearning process and the anxiety habituates. The stimulus loses its power to evoke distress.

Exposure therapy ameliorates the anxiety and emotional distress associated with OCD, whereas response prevention effectively reduces ritualizing. Both are necessary in treating most OCD patients (Foa et al. 1980a). A considerable amount of research has been devoted to establishing the treatment parameters for effective exposure and response prevention. The results largely parallel those obtained with the behavioral treatment of other anxiety disorders, such as panic with agoraphobia. Thus, it is possible for many OCD patients to master their symptoms more rapidly by practicing direct exposure to their most challenging, anxiety-provoking situations, a procedure known as *flooding*. Exposure therapy is a challenging treatment, however, and few patients are eager to pursue such an accelerated therapy. More typically, the therapist helps the patient construct a hierarchy of situations that elicit obsessions and rituals. The patient then practices mastering each item on the hierarchy in turn, developing a greater sense of self-efficacy and confidence with each step—a process termed *graded exposure therapy*.

The amount of time required for a patient to habituate to any given cue on his or her treatment hierarchy is variable, ranging from a few minutes to over 1 hour. The therapist, therefore, cannot be wed to the traditional 50-minute session. Early in treatment, moreover, it may be more helpful to conduct sessions two or three times per week. Exposure therapy usually begins with *imaginal exposure*, whereby the patient practices confronting the target situation in imagination before doing so in real life. The gains made during these visualizations pave the way for in vivo (i.e., real-life) exposure.

▌ Specific Behavioral Interventions

Although exposure and response prevention are the behavioral interventions best supported by empirical data, they are usually

implemented in the context of a more comprehensive, multimodal treatment plan. The following interventions, implemented in-
dividually or in groups, are those we have found most helpful.

Psychoeducation

Treatment begins by reviewing with the patient our current understanding of OCD and the role of behavior therapy and medication in its treatment. Patients are given reading material, such as
the pamphlets published by the Obsessive-Compulsive Foundation or one of several excellent self-help books, to examine and
share with their families. The notion of treatment as an active
partnership involving the development of self-management skills
is emphasized. This orientation is particularly important for those
individuals new to behavior therapy, since they may have been
accustomed to assuming a more passive role in medical treatment
or a less skills-oriented role in psychodynamic therapy. A brief
description and rationale is offered for each of the various components of behavioral treatment—such as exposure therapy, self-
monitoring, and home training—so that patients obtain a clear
view of the road ahead.

Self-Monitoring

During the first few weeks of treatment, patients are given special
forms and asked to keep a daily diary of their OCD symptoms.
They are asked to record the time of day that they experienced
symptoms, the situation that triggered them, the content of obsessive fears, and the duration or number of repetitions of rituals.
Self-monitoring is a valuable intervention on a number of levels.
It provides a baseline against which to measure progress. It also
serves as a rich source of information about the patient's unique
constellation of symptoms, triggering situations, and coping responses. Observations gleaned "in the heat of the moment" can
be more telling than the retrospective data obtained in the con-

fines of the therapist's office. Self-monitoring also offers a mechanism by which patients begin their transition from passive recipients of care to active participants in their own treatment. Keeping a daily diary fundamentally alters patients' relationships to their symptoms. Instead of perceiving themselves as powerless victims of mysterious, uncontrollable symptoms, they become interested observers of experiences that are relatively predictable, patterned, and mutable.

By actively observing their day-to-day experiences, of course, patients often discover new symptoms of which they had previously been only marginally aware. This heightened awareness, although enormously helpful, may initially demoralize some, who regard the additional symptoms as proof of even greater defectiveness and helplessness than they had supposed. It is important to help these patients to view such discoveries not as evidence of hopelessness but as invaluable information that will facilitate treatment.

Hierarchy Construction

Patients are helped to delineate each situation that elicits obsessive fears or urges to ritualize. Using a numerical rating scale of subjective units of distress (SUDS), they assign each situation a rating of 1 to 100 points, depending on how uncomfortable they would feel if they were unable to ritualize or to avoid that specific situation. The situations are mapped out with great clarity and are organized into a hierarchy ranging from the most easily managed to the most challenging ones. Separate hierarchies are constructed for each obsessional theme; for example, the same patient may require treatment for both contamination fears and concerns about harming someone. Each hierarchy typically includes 10–15 situations, although complex cases may require more, because treatment does not generalize very well to symptoms not specifically targeted. The increment in SUDS level (i.e., increase in discomfort) should be fairly consistent from one item in the hierarchy to the next.

Exposure Therapy and Response Prevention

Once the hierarchy has been constructed and the treatment process has been explained, the patient is usually ready to proceed with exposure and response prevention. The process often begins with imaginal exposure, as the patient is guided to imagine vividly a scene placed low on the hierarchy. To heighten the experience, the therapist coaches the patient to visualize concrete details about the setting (such as time of day, quality of the lighting, furniture in the room, color of clothing). The patient is then asked to focus on the specific anxiety-provoking cue, his or her obsessive fear, and his or her urges to ritualize or flee. A compulsive washer, for example, might be asked to imagine bringing a muddy shoe into the house, grasping the dirty sole in his hands, rubbing it against his skin, and grinding it into the pristinely clean carpet. The therapist sequentially draws attention to the patient's escalating emotional responses (anxiety, discomfort), cognitive reactions ("Oh Lord, this is contaminating everything!"), and physiological experiences (nausea, perspiration, racing heart), as well as to the patient's strong urges to ritualize or escape. The patient is encouraged to stay focused on the scene until the discomfort begins to abate. Periodically the therapist inquires as to the patient's SUDS level. Care must be taken to ensure that the patient does not distract him- or herself during the exposure trial by attending to other things, or try to counter the obsessive fears through subtle cognitive rituals that magically "undo" the perceived danger. When the SUDS level has diminished by 50%, the trial may be stopped. Dropping to a SUDS level at or below 20 is ideal but not essential. At each therapy session, the patient is guided through the same visualization. The patient is also asked to practice imagining this scene at home on a daily basis and to record his or her discomfort levels. He or she is instructed to refrain from ritualizing for a specified period of time following the exposure. Exposure trials at home and in therapy sessions continue until the scene no longer evokes discomfort. Treatment then moves on to the next hierarchy item.

Imaginal exposure helps set the stage for in vivo exposure,

which is a more powerful experience and a more critical focus of treatment. Imaginal work, however, takes on a greater importance for compulsive checkers, when the only practical way for the patient to confront fully his or her obsessive fears is through imagination. A patient who fears that the house will burn down if she doesn't ritualistically check that the stove is off, for example, can expose herself to this feared catastrophe only in imagination. In such cases, imaginal exposure to the feared future disaster (as opposed to only in vivo exposure to the situational cue) significantly enhances long-term treatment outcome (Foa et al. 1980b).

In vivo exposure to the target situation follows closely on the heels of imaginal exposure and is typically introduced in the same or a subsequent session. The patient is assisted to confront the triggering situation in real life, remaining fully in contact with it until the discomfort abates, without resorting to rituals or avoidance. (The patient who avoids dirt, for example, would be asked to bring a muddy shoe to the session and would practice rubbing it onto his hands, arms, face, and hair.) As with imaginal exposure, the therapist directs the patient's attention to his or her cognitive, affective, and physical responses to the obsessional cue, periodically assessing the patient's SUDS level until it has decreased by at least 50%. The patient practices exposure to that hierarchy item at home on a daily basis, recording his or her responses, until the situation no longer engenders discomfort. When necessary, the therapist models in vivo exposure for the patient (e.g., touching "contaminated" objects) before asking the patient to do the same. Research results suggest that "participant modeling" does not yield better clinical outcomes (Rachman et al. 1973), but many patients welcome it and it remains a common element of clinical practice.

Often, some or all of the patient's hierarchy items cannot be meaningfully addressed through in vivo exposure in the therapist's office because the relevant cues exist only in the home or in other real-world settings. For example, patients who compulsively check whether the lights are off and the door is locked before leaving home characteristically have no such concerns when leaving the therapist's office, since they are not gripped by the same oppressive sense of responsibility in that context. In these cases, the therapist cannot pursue in vivo exposure in his or her office. Depending on how refractory the symptoms are, the therapist may choose to accompany the patient into the appropriate setting, delegate a friend or relative to assist in the process, or encourage the patient to practice alone.

Response prevention is implemented in conjunction with exposure therapy. Patients are instructed to refrain from ritualizing in response to a specific hierarchy item, despite their strong impulses to the contrary. They are reminded that each time they ritualize, they inadvertently strengthen their OCD (via negative reinforcement), whereas resisting the rituals will become progressively easier with practice. Recommendations concerning how best to implement response prevention have varied widely in the literature, from the more permissive to the relatively draconian. Some treatment centers, for example, have addressed washing rituals by having the patient refrain from any washing for 2 hours following an exposure session (Baer and Minichiello 1990), while others have suspended *all* washing and showering for 5-day intervals (Steketee and Foa 1988). Response prevention seems to be a procedure of sufficient robustness that it remains effective despite considerable variations in technique, although some patients require firmer restrictions and oversight than others. In our own practice, we have found it helpful to instruct patients to refrain permanently from a given ritual once they have reached the associated target item in their hierarchies. If they are unable to stop completely, they work toward that goal through successive approximations, reducing the number of repetitions or increasing the duration of ritual-free intervals following exposure. Decreasing rituals very slowly is often harder than stopping them abruptly, however, and we encourage patients to eliminate each ritual as quickly as possible.

One of the great dangers of response prevention is that patients, wittingly or otherwise, may recruit ostensibly normal activities into the service of anxiety avoidance. Steketee and Foa (1988) carefully prohibit even "normal" hand washing and showering for compulsive cleaners early in treatment because these activities are so easily converted into a "decontaminating" exercise that would undermine treatment. Behaviors that can potentially be used to serve discomfort-relieving functions should be temporarily banned, even when they were not initially identified as "rituals." Along similar lines, patients sometimes develop covert cognitive rituals to make up for the absence of their overt behavioral rituals. Special words, repeated phrases, images, or prayers may be used to "undo" exposure to the upsetting cue. On the surface, it may appear that the patient is bravely adhering to the dictates of response prevention, and both therapist and patient may feel bewildered as to why treatment has suddenly plateaued. The presence of cognitive rituals should be assessed periodically throughout treatment. Finally, family members are often enlisted by the patient to fulfill rituals he or she has been prevented from performing. Ritualizing "by proxy" and compulsive requests to family members for reassurance (e.g., "Is the door *really* locked?") must be vigilantly identified and blocked.

Relaxation Training

In and of itself, relaxation training has not been helpful in ameliorating OCD symptoms. Indeed, it has often been used as a control condition in research studies to establish the efficacy of alternative treatments (e.g., Hodgson et al. 1972; Roper et al. 1975). OCD patients, however, often present with heightened levels of generalized anxiety. Relaxation training may be useful as an adjunctive strategy in lowering high baseline tension and arousal.

Unfortunately, OCD patients have a notoriously difficult time with relaxation procedures. As with trauma survivors or panic disorder patients, sitting still and focusing inward constitutes a tall order. Among the multiple types of relaxation strategies, those that offer a concrete task and a specific focus of attention, such as progressive muscle relaxation (Bernstein and Borkovec 1973), are often more accessible. Biofeedback devices such as inexpensive finger-held alcohol thermometers or electromyogram (EMG) instruments can also be helpful in vividly demonstrating to skeptical patients their capacity to have an impact on their own physiology. Many OCD patients profit from a brief course of relaxation training. Its role is clearly adjunctive, however, and if few gains are evident after a few sessions, therapy should not be detoured long toward a secondary intervention.

Cognitive Therapy

Cognitive interventions have traditionally been considered of little value in the treatment of OCD. To date, there are few empirical data on the subject. An often-cited early study (Emmelkamp et al. 1980) found no benefit in adding cognitive strategies (self-instructional training) to a standard package of exposure and response prevention, but a more recent study suggested promising results for rational emotive therapy, a more comprehensive approach (Emmelkamp et al. 1988). Heeding the literature's caveats, our clinic initially did not employ cognitive therapy strategies; over time, however, we have increasingly drawn on this modality in response to enthusiastic feedback from patients. The approaches we use—self-instructional training and cognitive restructuring—are similar to those adapted by Barlow and Cerny (1988) for use with panic disorder.

Self-instructional training stems from Donald Meichenbaum's work (1975, 1985). As applied to OCD treatment, such training is used to interrupt the crescendo of anxiety-provoking thoughts and images while replacing them with more grounding, task-focused cognitions. Patients are taught to examine the situations that elicit symptoms and to break them down into a series of smaller, more manageable stages. Specific stages include "preparing for the stressful situation," "confronting the stressful situation," "coping with feeling overwhelmed," and "evaluating the situation after it has passed." Patients are assisted in developing a set of coping self-statements for each stage to replace their automatic, self-defeating thoughts. They then practice coaching themselves through each stage using these positive self-statements. Patients record their coping statements on an index card, to which they can refer when practicing exposure therapy.

Cognitive restructuring (Beck and Emery 1985) is a more complex and elaborate approach. It seeks to fundamentally alter the way patients organize and process information about distressing situations instead of simply equipping them with self-soothing strategies. Patients are helped to become more attuned to their pattern of automatic, anxiety-provoking thoughts in situations that elicit OCD symptoms. They are then helped to gain distance from their automatic thoughts, and to assess the specific ways in which their interpretations are biased and distorted. Once patients have identified these "cognitive distortions," they are helped to generate more realistic, adaptive responses. In particular, therapy focuses on the tendency to overpredict catastrophic consequences, and the driving need for absolute certainty or completeness, that are hallmarks of OCD (Rasmussen and Eisen 1991).

By themselves, self-instructional training and cognitive restructuring probably have limited utility in the treatment of OCD. When combined with behavior therapy, however, these interventions can render symptoms more ego-dystonic and help patients to follow through with the rigors of exposure and response prevention. Patients who present with fixed ideas (overvalued ideation) about the necessity of their rituals and who respond less well to standard treatment sometimes benefit from cognitive interventions prior to attempting behavioral strategies.

Family Involvement

OCD has a profound impact on the patient's family. Over time, family life is often dramatically affected as relatives strive to understand, battle over, or accommodate—sometimes in astonishingly elaborate ways—the OCD patient's rituals and avoidance behavior. Families often feel bitter and resentful that their home life has become hostage to one member's panoply of symptoms. Ironically, the more they accommodate the patient's rituals and passive avoidance, the more entrenched the disorder becomes, because the patient is protected from exposure to his or her obsessional fears. Other patients, fearing humiliation or rejection, struggle valiantly to keep their OCD secret from other family members, thereby cultivating the seeds of alienation.

Because OCD can become so tenaciously woven into the fabric of family life, it is enormously helpful to involve the family in treatment. It is therefore striking that family dynamics and therapy have thus far received relatively scant attention in the adult treatment literature, notwithstanding some innovative work with multiple family groups at Brown University (Van Noppen et al. 1991; also see Cobb et al. 1980). In our own clinic, families are initially provided with basic education about the disorder and are offered reading material. Common emotional reactions such as confusion, anger, bewilderment, and self-blame, often long-simmering but unexpressed, are processed and normalized. The treatment rationale and interventions are reviewed with family members and their support solicited. Discussions also focus on the dangers of inadvertently reinforcing the patient's symptoms by participating in rituals, responding to his or her frequent requests for reassurance, or facilitating his or her avoidance of feared situations (e.g., family members removing shoes and clothes before entering the house to prevent "contamination" of the home). If the family is supportive, relatives can be enlisted as "coaches" to assist the patient in home training. The additional structure and support that such assistance affords the patient can be an invaluable asset, sometimes making the difference between successful and unsuccessful outpatient treatment. Families are also encouraged to participate in one of the growing number of community-based OCD support groups that have become available in recent years (the Obsessive-Compulsive Foundation is a helpful resource is locating these services).

Relapse Prevention Training

Typically, relapse prevention is thought of as an intervention employed at the end of treatment to help patients maintain gains and to inoculate them against future setbacks. We have found it important to include relapse-prevention principles from the very beginning of treatment, and these principles color the manner in which all self-management tools and skills are presented. Complex change is rarely a simple, linear progression. Slips and setbacks are intrinsic to the process. Anxious patients, particularly those with OCD, tend to develop rigidly polarized, black-and-white perceptions of themselves and the world. They are prone to view setbacks as catastrophic and immutable failures, and to become highly skeptical or demoralized as a result. It is extremely important to help OCD patients prepare themselves in advance to experience slips and to work through the meaning of these experiences in more adaptive, less cataclysmic terms. Patients are helped to understand that some setbacks are inevitable, and that during times of stress they will be particularly vulnerable to symptom recurrence. Most importantly, they are helped to view slips as valuable learning opportunities rather than signposts of defeat. They are taught to carefully analyze their experiences to discover what factors may have contributed to the slip, and how they can better cope with such circumstances in the future (Marlatt 1985). Toward the end of treatment, we sometimes have patients practice coping with a "relapse" by intentionally reintroducing a previously mastered symptom. The experience of successfully re-eliminating the obsession or ritual builds patients' confidence that they can manage effectively in the future.

▌ Treatment Modalities and the Therapist's Role in Behavior Therapy

In uncomplicated cases, behavior therapy for OCD is usually administered over the course of 15–20 sessions of active treatment, with a few periodic booster sessions during the maintenance phase. Individual therapy is the norm in most clinics, but we have become increasingly convinced of the value of a specialized group program, which we began developing in 1988 (A. Sherman, "Behavioral Group Therapy for Obsessive-Compulsive Disorder: A Treatment Manual" [unpublished manuscript], September 1988). Groups are a particularly appropriate format for OCD patients because they help counter the debilitating sense of isolation and shame characteristic of the disorder. Most patients find it an eye-opening experience to meet others who have wrestled with similar difficulties. Groups help legitimize the struggles patients have had with OCD and nurture them through the hurdles of a demanding treatment. In our groups, patients are encouraged to establish a "buddy system" during the initial phase of the 15-week program. Subsequently, buddies accompany each other on "field trips" to relevant settings, where they assist each other in practicing exposure and response prevention until they are able to handle these situations independently. Aside from providing additional structure, groups thus present participants with an opportunity to be helpful to others, itself an empowering experience. These activities help salvage badly battered self-esteem and challenge the self-representation of being utterly powerless in the face of OCD. In these days of managed care, it is also worth exploring whether group treatment may be more cost-effective than individual therapy.

As a rule, cognitive-behavior therapy calls for a therapist who is comfortable with an active, directive, warmly collaborative posture. With OCD, the patient's tendency toward avoidance can be so gripping and compelling that a stronger dose of clarity and firmness is often required on the part of the therapist (Steketee and Tynes 1991). Therapists who are highly permissive and accommodating tend not to fare well in terms of treatment outcome, relative to those who are more challenging and explicit (Rabavilas et al. 1979). The types of transference issues that are apt to unfold over the course of behavioral treatment are highly variable; consistent with some of the classic psychodynamic literature, issues concerning control and narcissistic vulnerability are not uncommon, perhaps intensified by a demanding therapy. Although a focus on transference is not viewed as the primary agent of change, these issues should be addressed to the extent that they impede treatment adherence or progress.

Interestingly, there is now a move toward greater reliance upon self-directed treatment in the anxiety disorders. As with agoraphobia, social phobias, and specific phobias (see Marks 1987), it seems clear that a number of OCD patients can successfully pursue exposure therapy on their own, with limited therapist involvement, once they have been properly trained in the techniques (Emmelkamp and van Kraanen 1977; Marks et al. 1988). This specific, systematic training stands in marked contrast to informal encouragement of patients simply to confront the situations that upset them. As emphasized by Marks and colleagues (1988), "the process involved is far from a glib exercise in telling them to 'use willpower to face the fear.' Very few cases respond to such simplistic advice" (p. 532). Whether particular subgroups of patients best suited for self-guided treatment can be identified remains to be investigated empirically.

■ Caveats and Contraindications for Behavior Therapy

Although behavior therapy for OCD has led to substantial gains across controlled outcome studies, it is not without salient drawbacks. It is a challenging, anxiety-provoking treatment that requires a significant commitment of time and energy for its success. Increasingly, attention has focused on what kinds of patients respond most and least favorably. Some of the variables considered predictive of poor outcome with behavioral treatment have been highlighted by Baer and Minichiello (1990) and Foa (1979). Rudimentary guidelines have been discussed for many years, but subsequent research has not always supported these assumptions. From our own vantage point, working with a large number of patients who manifest severe psychopathology, we regard these variables more as caveats than strong contraindications. Patients possessing problematic characteristics do require more judicious attention to transference issues, pacing of treatment, adjunctive services, and social supports.

Poor compliance with treatment is one common reason for failure. This is hardly surprising given the emphasis placed by behavior therapy on developing tools and practicing self-management skills. There are innumerable reasons for poor adherence, however, and such behavior should be taken as a starting point for exploration with the patient rather than as a fixed indicator of impending failure. Severe depression has typically been regarded as a contraindication for exposure therapy. Depression is of course a frequent complication of OCD, but severely depressed patients tend not to habituate despite prolonged exposure to the feared situation (Foa et al. 1982, 1983; Marks 1981). It is also more difficult for such patients to follow through with the active home practice sessions and self-monitoring requirements. Thus, severe depression should be attended to prior to initiating exposure and response prevention. Moderate levels of depression, however, are not in general an impediment (Cottraux et al. 1990; Marks et al. 1988).

Behavioral treatment has also been widely considered to be less effective in patients with overvalued ideation (Foa 1979), although not all studies have borne out this assumption (Foa et al. 1983). In contrast to those who recognize that their ritualizing is irrational, patients with ego-syntonic, fixed beliefs about the necessity for their rituals probably will not respond well, both because the goal of treatment is perceived as highly dissonant and because their overall level of functioning is usually more compromised. Cognitive approaches, concretely implemented, are sometimes helpful as a first-stage intervention in rendering these patients' symptoms more dystonic and amenable to subsequent behavioral work. We almost invariably provide these patients, too, with pharmacotherapy.

Along similar lines, patients with schizotypal personality disorder are often poorer candidates for both standard behavioral and pharmacological treatment (Minichiello et al. 1987). As noted by Baer and Minichiello (1990), such individuals often embody most of the poor prognostic indicators outlined above, with their proclivities toward poor treatment adherence, impoverished interpersonal relationships, overvalued ideation, and magical thinking. One investigation found no significant relationship between personality disorders and treatment outcome (Steketee 1988); however, our experience concurs with that of others who have observed that patients with fixed beliefs, magical thinking, marginal interpersonal functioning, and low-level thought disorder, presenting across a spectrum of psychopathology ranging from schizotypal to "schizo-obsessive" or "obsessive psychotic," are decidedly more difficult to treat (Baer and Minichiello 1990; Rachman and Hodgson 1980). Developing more effective interventions for these patients remains a major challenge.

Special treatment considerations also apply to certain subtypes of OCD. Patients who have obsessions without overt rituals, for example, are often presumed to be less responsive to behavior therapy. There is some empirical evidence that this is the case (Christensen et al. 1987)—and, indeed, most outcome research on behavioral treatment has conscientiously excluded this subtype of OCD. Nevertheless, it is not clear that patients with "pure obsessions" (often incorrectly categorized, since many have cognitive rituals as well) are as treatment refractory as has been assumed. The traditional behavioral intervention for obsessions without overt rituals has been thought stopping, a technique intended to interrupt the flow of intrusive cognitions. This strategy is easy to teach patients but has yielded mixed results (Emmelkamp and Kwee 1977; Stern 1978). However, studies employing careful, systematic exposure to the obsessional thoughts—for example, by exposing patients to a continuous tape-recording of their upsetting thoughts while blocking neutralizing cognitive rituals—have demonstrated very promising results (Hoogduin et al. 1987; Salkovskiis and Westbrook 1989). In our clinic, we offer patients with "pure obsessions" a brief trial of thought stopping, followed if needed by exposure therapy. Pharmacotherapy, too, is often an important treatment component (Volavka et al. 1985). Additional interventions might include cognitive restructuring or mindfulness meditation.

Another category of patients considered less responsive to treatment includes those with primary obsessional slowness. These individuals' consuming preoccupation with precision, symmetry, and aligning things "just right" means that even simple tasks require an extraordinary amount of time for completion (Rasmussen and Eisen 1991). Although exasperating to others, these symptoms are not regarded as particularly disturbing or unreasonable by the patients. There are no special feared disasters associated with functioning in a normal, nonritualized manner, but rather a general, progressively mounting sense of tension. Behavior therapy for these patients involves systematically and concretely guiding them as they complete specific tasks within contracted periods of time. The process of coaching such individuals through successive approximations is slow-going and requires considerable structure and patience (Baer and Minichiello 1990).

▌ Pharmacotherapy: An Overview of Current Approaches

Some of the most exciting and rapidly growing areas of research in OCD concern the search for underlying biological mechanisms and extrapolation of pharmacotherapeutic strategies. Family pedigree studies, although compromised by methodological limitations, have suggested that up to 25% of first-degree relatives of OCD subjects have subclinical OCD features themselves (e.g., Swedo et al. 1989). Similarly, twin studies have found a higher concordance rate for OCD in identical than in nonidentical twins (Liebowitz and Hollander 1991; Rasmussen and Eisen 1990). These data suggest a partial role for genetic transmission, particularly for a subset of OCD patients. The most intriguing findings, however, have come from biochemical and neuroanatomical studies. Preliminary evidence from these separate lines of investigation suggests dysfunction in the frontal lobe–anterior cingulate–basal ganglia circuit, driven by impairment in the striatum (Baxter et al. 1991). Imaging studies continue to explore this possibility.

OCD has been correlated with an increase in the activity of serotonergic brain pathways (Zohar and Insel 1987), although dopamine may play a role as well (Goodman et al. 1990a). Serotonin's importance is suggested, for example, by the observation that OCD symptoms worsen under experimental conditions that temporarily increase postsynaptic serotonergic activity, such as some of the pharmacological challenge studies using the serotonin agonist *m*-chlorophenylpiperazine (mCPP) (Hollander et al. 1988; Zohar et al. 1987). In addition, clinicians have noted that the medications most effective in treating OCD are those that more or less selectively block serotonin synaptic reuptake. Although the mechanism remains incompletely elucidated, effective sustained treatment appears to decrease the activity of these pathways, perhaps by downregulating the activity of postsynaptic receptors or by stimulating the self-inhibiting activity of the presynaptic neurons. Positron-emission tomography (PET) studies consistent with this hypothesis have demonstrated changes in serotonergic activity in the orbital gyri and striatal areas (Baxter et al. 1990); furthermore, the changes produced by effective treatment may be similar regardless of whether that treatment is pharmacological or behavioral (Baxter et al. 1992).

The pharmacotherapy of OCD is usually straightforward, although a significant minority of patients do not respond to an initial medication trial (Goodman et al. 1992) and some patients do not respond at all. An active medication is necessary since OCD sufferers tend not to respond to placebo treatment (Mavissakalian et al. 1990). In contrast to patients with panic disorder or depression, OCD patients often require a longer duration of pharmacotherapy in order to fully assess therapeutic response. A trial of 10–12 weeks may be necessary to avoid prematurely labeling a medication regimen ineffective (Jenike 1991). Clinical experience suggests also that, relative to the pharmacotherapy of panic disorder or depression, OCD treatment requires higher dosages. Unfortunately, there is as yet little empirical evidence to substantiate this impression (see Greist et al. [1992], Tollefson et al. [1994], and Wheadon [1991] for disconfirming data), and further studies are required to distinguish effects of dose from those of treatment duration for each medication (Goodman et al. 1992).

Several antidepressants that increase the synaptic availability of serotonin by blocking its presynaptic reuptake or reabsorption from the synapse have been shown to be effective in treating both obsessions and compulsions. Although classified as "antidepressants," these medications have antiobsessional effects that are independent of their antidepressant effects. Clomipramine, a tricylic antidepressant with potent serotonin reuptake inhibiting properties, has been demonstrated to be superior both to placebo and to several tricyclic antidepressants (TCAs) in a number of studies (Ananth et al. 1981; Clomipramine Collaborative Study Group 1991; Insel et al. 1983; Jaskari 1980; Mavissakalian et al. 1985; Montgomery 1980; Thorén et al. 1980; Volavka et al. 1985; Zohar and Insel 1987). Improvement is estimated to occur in 50%–66% of patients treated (Clomipramine Collaborative Study Group 1991; Zohar et al. 1992). Clomipramine is usually begun in OCD patients at a dosage of 25 mg po qhs, and then increased to a maximum trial dose that produces a serum level of 300–350 ng/ml. Such a dose is usually about 200–250 mg/day. Although clomipramine is the most extensively studied and empirically validated medication for OCD, it is often associated with bothersome side effects (Pigott et al. 1990). Sedation, anticholinergic dry mouth and constipation, dizziness, orthostatic hypotension, and weight gain are side effects that patients find particularly troubling. Anorgasmia may be more of a problem than is generally recognized, because patients are reluctant to report it (Monteiro et al. 1987).

Side effects typically emerge before clinical improvement occurs and thus can potentially undermine patient compliance. Compliance can be enhanced, however, by educating patients carefully about the anticipated beneficial and adverse effects of treatment. Sedation can often be managed by dosing at bedtime. Constipation can be reduced by recommending increased fluid intake and dietary fiber and, if necessary, prescribing a stool softener (Pato and Zohar 1991). Difficulties with dizziness or blurred vision usually dissipate after the first few weeks of treatment (Stern et al. 1980).

Other antidepressants with more specific effects on serotonergic activity—the SSRIs—have also shown results roughly comparable to those obtained with clomipramine, with less extensive side effects. Preliminary controlled trials have suggested efficacy for fluoxetine (Pigott et al. 1990; Turner et al. 1985), sertraline (Chouinard et al. 1990), and fluvoxamine (Goodman et al. 1989a, 1990b; Jenike et al. 1990; Perse et al. 1987). Anecdotally, paroxetine also appears effective. Studies are currently under way to compare the relative efficacies of these agents. Fluoxetine is often started at a dosage of 10–20 mg/day and increased to 20–60 mg/day (Tollefson et al. 1994). For a few patients, it may be necessary to use a large daily dosage, typically 60–80 mg/day. The maximal response may not be achieved for several months. Although often better tolerated than clomipramine, fluoxetine has a spectrum of side effects that include restlessness, nausea, loss of appetite, and impaired sexual function. Sertraline is begun at 25 or 50 mg/day and increased to a maximum of 200 mg/day, whereas paroxetine is started at 20 mg/day and increased to 40 or 60 mg/day. These drugs possess a spectrum of side effects that is similar to fluoxetine's, although the frequency of any particular adverse reaction may differ with each drug.

When patients fail to respond to initial monotherapy (treatment with a single medication) or find that medication's side effects intolerable, another serotonin-enhancing antidepressant can be tried. As an alternative or further treatment approach, a variety of augmentation strategies have been proposed, using agents that are ir.effective independently but may be helpful in conjunction with a serotonergic antidepressant. Psychopharmacologists at Yale University School of Medicine (Goodman et al. 1992) and Harvard Medical School (Jenike 1991) have developed algorithms, based largely on clinical experience, to help guide decision making in this area. Although not yet empirically validated, these schemes provide useful preliminary guidelines for clinical practice.

To begin with, insufficient response to either clomipramine or an SSRI should suggest a trial of the alternate agent. In some cases, an SSRI can even be combined with clomipramine (Zetin and Kramer 1992) to arrive at an effective treatment regimen with a side-effect profile tailored to an individual patient's tolerance. Goodman and colleagues (1992) recommend proceeding to a second SSRI trial when an initial one has failed. If improvement has been unsatisfactory yet side effects are tolerable through two consecutive SSRI trials, augmentation with another agent is recommended.

Buspirone, for example, is a serotonin-enhancing anxiolytic

usually employed in the treatment of generalized anxiety disorder that has been combined with antidepressants in treating OCD (Jenike 1990a; Zetin and Kramer 1992). The results of buspirone trials have been inconsistent, although some positive responses have been documented (Jenike et al. 1991; McDougle et al. 1993a). A trial of buspirone augmentation can begin at 5 mg bid with a gradual increase to 10 mg qid, although even larger dosages have been used with some patients. Lithium augmentation, although perhaps capable of enhancing medication response in patients with a concurrent mood disorder, has also led to inconsistent results when subjected to controlled observation (McDougle et al. 1993b; Rasmussen 1984). This strategy should be employed cautiously (Jenike 1991) in light of the reported potential for lithium toxicity in conjunction with fluoxetine treatment (Noveske et al. 1989; Salama and Shafey 1989).

For several special categories of patients, adjunctive treatment can be particularly useful. OCD patients with schizotypal features or delusion-like obsessions often benefit from adjunctive neuroleptic treatment (Jenike 1990a; Zetin and Kramer 1992). In one study (McDougle et al. 1990), OCD patients with chronic tics or schizotypal personality disorder showed a superior response when a neuroleptic was added to fluvoxamine treatment. Adjunctive clonazepam or a switch to MAOI treatment has been suggested for patients with comorbid panic disorder. MAOI pharmacotherapy has been advocated for patients who suffer from obsessions without compulsions (Jenike 1990a). Because of the potential for highly toxic and even fatal drug interactions, however, discontinuation of the SSRI must precede MAOI treatment. Discontinuation of fluoxetine 5 weeks in advance of MAOI treatment is recommended, whereas a minimum of 2 weeks' advance discontinuation is recommended for treatment with one of the other serotonin-enhancing drugs (Dista Products 1988; Jenike 1991; Sternback 1988).

For patients who show little or no response to several trials of pharmacotherapy, with or without concurrent behavior therapy, reconsideration of the primary diagnosis may be indicated. A common obstacle to effective treatment response is the failure to take into account a comorbid psychiatric disorder such as schizotypal personality disorder, substance abuse, depression, schizophrenia, or an organic mental disorder (Zetin and Kramer 1992). Ongoing psychosocial stressors must be reassessed, too, to determine their role in prolonging or exacerbating OCD symptoms. Finally, evidence of the patient's compliance with medication dosage instructions should be sought.

▌ Integrating Behavior Therapy and Pharmacotherapy for OCD

Given the importance of combining or selecting between behavioral and pharmacological treatments for anxiety disorders in everyday clinical practice, it is surprising and disheartening that so few empirical data are available to guide decisions. In practice, decisions to offer behavioral treatment or medication are often shaped more by the proclivities, resources, and biases of the treating clinician than by a thoughtful consideration of applicable alternatives. It is clear that each modality is a viable treatment for many patients. The respective bodies of outcome research suggest somewhat comparable clinical efficacies. Roughly 50%–65% of patients who remain in treatment with clomipramine significantly benefit, with an average improvement rate of about 40% (Abel 1993; Clomipramine Collaborative Study Group 1991; Goodman et al. 1992; Greist 1990; Spiegel 1992). Approximately 70%–90% of patients who remain in treatment with behavior therapy significantly improve, with perhaps a 60% average improvement rate (Foa et al. 1985; Marks et al. 1988; Spiegel 1992). The number of patients who decline to start treatment or who subsequently drop out varies from roughly 10% to 25% for both behavioral treatment (Foa et al. 1983, 1984; Marks et al. 1988; Rachman and Hodgson 1980) and clomipramine (DeVeaugh-Geiss et al. 1989; Marks et al. 1988; Mavissakalian et al. 1990; Volavka et al. 1985). In our experience, adherence is somewhat better for pharmacotherapy, although the opposite view has also been proposed (Marks et al. 1988). Contrasting these data involves comparing "apples and or-

anges," since most of the studies from which they are derived involve differently constituted samples and differing research de-
signs; however, the consistency of results across investigations
adds a measure of credibility. There is a pressing need for more
controlled comparison studies.

Much of the controlled comparison research that does exist is
compromised by methodological limitations that undermine the
generalizability of results to actual clinical practice. The work of
Marks and colleagues is among the most sophisticated in this area
and therefore deserves further discussion. In an initial study
(Marks et al. 1980), 40 moderately depressed OCD patients were
randomly assigned to receive either clomipramine or placebo.
Each of these groups was in turn divided, so that half of each pharmacotherapy group received 15 sessions of inpatient exposure
therapy and response prevention, while the other half received
15 sessions of relaxation training (i.e., psychological placebo). After 7 weeks of medication (or placebo) combined with 3 weeks of
behavioral treatment, those who received clomipramine were significantly more improved than those who received placebo. Those
who received exposure therapy had improved to a significantly
greater degree than those who received relaxation training. The
combination of clomipramine and exposure therapy was superior
to either treatment alone. As the study continued, the combination
of clomipramine and exposure therapy remained more effective
than exposure therapy alone, although this difference in effectiveness was no longer statistically reliable at the end of 1 year. The
superiority of the combined treatment in this study, however, was
attributable to the gains made by very depressed patients. Subjects
who were less depressed were not shown to benefit significantly
from the addition of clomipramine to behavior therapy.

A number of other authorities, however, have questioned the
generalizability of this conclusion. The Marks et al. (1980) study
has been criticized for using rather low doses of clomipramine,
perhaps reducing the effectiveness of the pharmacotherapy trial,
although the authors stated that dosages were as high as patients
would tolerate. Furthermore, the brevity of the period from which
data were drawn to compare clomipramine alone with behavior

therapy alone appears to underrepresent the potency of either treatment. Finally, most other studies have found a specific antiobsessional effect for clomipramine that is independent of level of depression (e.g., Insel et al. 1983; Mavissakalian et al. 1985; Thorén et al. 1980).

A subsequent study by Marks and colleagues (1988) was designed to provide further information concerning the value of combining exposure therapy with clomipramine treatment. Previous research had failed to control for the helpful effect of the informal, self-guided exposure to upsetting situations that was typically recommended to pharmacotherapy patients. To more effectively control for the influence of this confounding factor, 44 OCD subjects were randomly assigned to receive 1) clomipramine with explicit instructions to avoid anxiety-provoking exposure and response prevention (i.e., "anti-exposure instructions"), 2) clomipramine with self-guided exposure therapy, 3) clomipramine with both self-guided and therapist-guided exposure therapies, or 4) placebo with self- and therapist-guided exposure therapies. After 8 weeks, clomipramine with self-guided exposure was superior to self-guided exposure alone. These differences did not, however, persist throughout the 6-month treatment period and subsequent 6-month follow-up period. Exposure therapy proved equally effective with or without the addition of clomipramine. A finding of great interest was that patients who received clomipramine and who were told to avoid exposure to anxiety-provoking situations did so poorly that more than half were removed from that part of the study 5 weeks early. These results suggest that any pharmacotherapy patient should routinely receive a recommendation to confront rather than avoid upsetting stimuli. Spiegel (1992), in particular, has speculated that "the main value of the serotonin reuptake inhibitors in OCD may lie in their ability to make it easier for patients to confront the things they avoid. Without such exposure, the utility of the drugs is questionable" (p. 2). Data consistent with that conclusion have also been obtained with imipramine, used in the treatment of agoraphobic patients who were instructed to *avoid* exposure to anxiety-provoking situations (Telch et al. 1985).

A subsequent study by Cottraux and colleagues (1990) com-

pared fluvoxamine treatment and exposure therapy and found
similar results. Sixty moderately depressed OCD patients were
randomly assigned to fluvoxamine with antiexposure instructions,
fluvoxamine with exposure therapy, or placebo with exposure
therapy. Unfortunately, the antiexposure condition was invali-
dated by a number of factors: patient compliance was very poor,
several patients dropped out because they were so dissatisfied with
this treatment, and some of the instructions inadvertently mixed
aspects of exposure with antiexposure. After 8 weeks, the ritualizing of subjects in each of the three treatment conditions had significantly improved. There was a temporary superiority for
fluvoxamine over placebo on one of nine ritual measures. By the
end of 24 weeks of treatment, each group had continued to improve, and all treatments were comparably effective in reducing
rituals. These gains were maintained at 6-month follow-up. The
percentage of patients classified as "improved" in their OCD suggested an advantage for the combined treatment, but these differences were not statistically reliable. Thus, the results of this study
echo those of Marks and colleagues (1988), showing no definitive
long-term advantage for adding an SSRI to exposure therapy.

It remains tempting on the basis of clinical experience, nonetheless, to assume that the integration of behavioral treatment and
pharmacotherapy has more to offer than either treatment alone.
The results of the studies noted here, however, as well as the findings of other, methodologically more limited studies, do not un-
ambiguously answer clinicians' questions on this matter. Further
research, examining the effects of separate and combined treatments in large samples over a sufficiently long interval, with sufficiently high medication dosages, is clearly needed.

While we await further research findings, a variety of considerations support the use of integrated treatment. Each intervention
appears helpful where the other is weakest. The addition of an
SSRI to behavior therapy is apt to improve compliance with what
patients consider a rigorous enterprise (Marks et al. 1980). It may
also lead to faster gains in the short term (Cottraux et al. 1990;
Marks et al. 1988), notwithstanding the sometimes slower antiobsessional effects of SSRIs relative to their antidepressant effects.

The addition of an SSRI is also more effective in improving mood, a particularly important consideration with severely depressed OCD patients (Cottraux et al. 1990; Foa et al. 1982, 1983; Marks 1981). Those with overvalued ideation are apt to do better with concurrent medication than with behavioral treatment alone (Foa 1979). Finally, even though its success is often limited (Minichiello et al. 1987), pharmacotherapy is probably more effective in treating patients with relatively severe comorbid Axis I or Axis II psychopathology and ego-syntonic OCD symptoms. Preliminary data suggest that fluoxetine (Baer and Jenike 1990), but not clomipramine (Baer et al. 1992), is helpful in treating OCD in patients with comorbid schizotypal, paranoid, or schizoid personality disorders. Anecdotally, we have certainly seen many patients with severe character disorders or subtle psychotic symptoms who were able to make some use of behavioral treatment only after they were placed on appropriate regimens of neuroleptics and/or SSRIs.

Conversely, the addition of behavioral treatment to pharmacotherapy tends to redress one of the most serious drawbacks of unimodal pharmacotherapy of OCD—the inordinately high relapse rate. Relapse rates in controlled studies that combined the two treatments were notably low (Cottraux et al. 1990; Marks et al. 1988). Cost savings could reasonably be expected from employment of integrated treatment, notwithstanding the initial heightened expense for two treatments, if patients are subsequently able to avoid the expenses associated with extremely long-term medication regimens. Further, as noted above, it is possible that the efficacy of medication treatment relies to some extent on exposure to anxiety-provoking cues, whether pursued systematically or incidentally. If so, formal behavior therapy would be expected to facilitate the pharmacotherapy process. Finally, the addition of behavior therapy to pharmacotherapy may provide psychological benefits by instilling a sense of mastery and self-efficacy that medication alone usually fails to confer. Patients who have worked through a course of cognitive-behavioral treatment typically come away with a heightened appreciation of their own resources and capacities. This shift in self-representation is an important aspect of their experience. Adding behavior therapy to pharmacotherapy may foster this kind of evolution, provided that the caregivers can assist OCD patients to avoid attributing all gains to their medications. Finally, patients with severe concomitant psychopathology who respond only partially to medications may benefit to a greater degree from the addition of behavioral and supportive treatments, modified according to their special needs, with emphasis on slower pacing, more extensive structure, and additional social supports.

Some OCD patients express clear preferences for either behavior therapy or medication, or are deemed inappropriate candidates for one or the other treatment. Most patients, however, are amenable to integrated treatment and seem to profit from the advantages of this approach. In clinical practice, integrated treatment usually entails a collaboration between a prescribing physician and a behavior therapist. OCD patients often readily accept the involvement of a team approach and feel reassured at the prospect of two professionals assisting them with their difficulties. Assuming the requisite level of cooperation, communication, and clarity of roles between prescribing physician and therapist, few problems are encountered in coordinating care.

▌ Conclusions

Current treatmants for OCD offer patients brighter prospects for recovery, reduced suffering, and improved quality of life than have previously been attainable. In this chapter we have reviewed some of the important elements of cognitive-behavioral and pharmacological treatments for OCD and discussed the potential value of integrating these approaches.

In clinical practice, integrated treatment implies more than a simple combination of distinct interventions. Integrated care requires a mutually established treatment plan, clear roles, close coordination, and a genuine spirit of collaboration. Without this type of partnership, combined treatments can inadvertently undermine each other. For example, a psychopharmacologist's focus on bio-chemical factors may leave patients skeptical that psychosocial fac-tors or learned patterns of avoidance have any place in their difficulties. Conversely, the treatment rationale offered by a cog-nitive-behavior therapist may devalue the role of medication.

Further research is required to confirm whether, and for which patients, integrated treatment may be more helpful than single treatments for OCD. Our clinical experience is that integrated care has much to offer. Relative to pharmacotherapy alone, inte-grated treatment may provide many patients with a new range of coping skills (with positive effects in other areas of life), reduced feelings of helplessness, and significantly lower relapse rates. Rela-tive to cognitive-behavior therapy alone, it may offer many pa-tients more rapid onset of symptom relief, greater tolerance for and compliance with exposure therapy, and more reliable reduc-tion in comcomitant depression. Patients with severe comorbid pathology may also respond better to appropriately designed inte-grated therapy than to unimodal interventions. Investigations are beginning to explore these issues. In the interim, OCD patients will be best served if their clinicians are sensitive to the advantages that each of these treatments can provide.

▮ References

Abel JL: Exposure with response prevention and serotonergic an-tidepressants in the treatment of obsessive-compulsive disorder: a review and implications for interdisciplinary treatment. Behav Res Ther 31:463–478, 1993

American Psychiatric Association: Diagnostic and Statistical Man-ual of Mental Disorders, 4th Edition. Washington, DC, Ameri-can Psychiatric Association, 1994

Ananth J, Pecknold JC, van den Steen N, et al: Double-blind com-parative study of clomipramine and amitriptyline in obsessive neurosis. Progress in Neuro-Psychopharmacology 5:257–262, 1981

Baer L, Jenike MA: Personality disorders in obsessive-compulsive disorder, in Obsessive-Compulsive Disorders: Theory and Management, 2nd Edition. Edited by Jenike MA, Baer L, Minichiello WE. Chicago, IL, Year Book Medical, 1990, pp 84–85

Baer L, Jenike MA, Black DW, et al: Effect of Axis II diagnoses on treatment outcome with clomipramine in 54 patients with obsessive-compulsive disorder. Arch Gen Psychiatry 49:862–866, 1992

Baer L, Jenike MA, Ricciari JN, et al: Standardized assessment of personality disorders in obsessive-compulsive disorder. Arch Gen Psychiatry 47:826–830, 1990

Baer L, Minichiello WE: Behavior therapy for obsessive-compulsive disorder, in Obsessive-Compulsive Disorders: Theory and Management, 2nd Edition. Edited by Jenike MA, Baer L, Minichiello WE. Chicago, IL, Year Book Medical, 1990, pp 203–232

Barlow DH, Cerny JA: Cognitive treatment component, in Psychological Treatment of Panic. New York, Guilford, 1988, pp 120–150

Barlow DH, DiNardo PA, Vermilyea BB: Comorbidity and depression among the anxiety disorders. J Nerv Ment Dis 174:63–72, 1986

Baxter LR, Schwartz JM, Bergman KS, et al: Caudate glucose metabolic changes with both drug and behavior therapy for obsessive-compulsive disorder. Arch Gen Psychiatry 49:681–689, 1992

Baxter LR, Schwartz JM, Gruz BH: Brain imaging: toward a neuroanatomy of OCD, in The Psychobiology of Obsessive-Compulsive Disorder. Edited by Zohar J, Insel T, Rasmussen S. New York, Springer, 1991, pp 101–125

Baxter LR, Schwartz JM, Guze BH, et al: PET imaging in obsessive-compulsive disorder with and without depression. J Clin Psychiatry 51 (suppl):61–69, 1990

Beck AT, Emery G: Anxiety Disorders and Phobias: A Cognitive Perspective. New York, Basic Books, 1985

Bernstein DA, Borkovec TD: Progressive Relaxation Training: A Manual for the Helping Professions. Champaign, IL, Research Press, 1973

Boulougouris JC, Bassiakos L: Prolonged flooding in cases with obsessive-compulsive neurosis. Behav Res Ther 11:227–231, 1973

Chouinard G, Goodman W, Greist J, et al: Results of a double-blind placebo-controlled trial of a new serotonin uptake inhibitor, sertraline, in the treatment of obsessive-compulsive disorder. Psychopharmacol Bull 26:279–284, 1990

Christensen H, Hadzi-Pavlovic K, Andrews G, et al: Behavior therapy and tricylic medication in the treatment of obsessive-compulsive disorder: a quantitative review. J Consult Clin Psychol 55:701–711, 1987

Clomipramine Collaborative Study Group: Clomipramine in the treatment of patients with obsessive-compulsive disorder. Arch Gen Psychiatry 48:730–738, 1991

Cobb JP, McDonald R, Marks IM, et al: Marital versus exposure therapy: psychological treatments of coexisting marital and phobic-obsessive problems. Behavioural Analysis and Modification 4:3–16, 1980

Cottraux J, Mollard E, Bouvard M, et al: A controlled study of fluvoxamine and exposure in obsessive-compulsive disorder. Int Clin Psychopharmacol 5:17–30, 1990

DeVeaugh-Geiss J, Landau P, Katz R: Preliminary results from a multicenter trial of clomipramine in obsessive-compulsive disorder. Psychopharmacol Bull 25:36–40, 1989

Dista Products: Prozac: Comprehensive Monograph. Indianapolis, IN, Eli Lilly & Company, 1988

Emmelkamp PMG, Kwee KG: Obsessional ruminations: a comparison between thought stopping and prolonged exposure in imagination. Behav Res Ther 15:441–444, 1977

Emmelkamp PMG, van Kraanen J: Therapist-controlled exposure in vivo: a comparison with obsessive-compulsive patients. Behav Res Ther 15:491–495, 1977

Emmelkamp PMG, van der Helm M, van Zanten BL, et al: Contributions of self-instructional training to the effectiveness of exposure in vivo: a comparison with obsessive-compulsive patients. Behav Res Ther 18:61–66, 1980

Emmelkamp PMG, Viser S, Hoekstra RJ: Cognitive therapy vs. exposure in vivo in the treatment of obsessive-compulsives. Cognitive Therapy and Research 12:103–114, 1988

Foa EB: Failure in treating obsessive-compulsives. Behav Res Ther 17:169–176, 1979

Foa EB, Goldstein A: Continuous exposure and complete response prevention of obsessive-compulsive disorder. Behavior Therapy 9:821–829, 1978

Foa EB, Steketee GS, Milby JB: Differential effects of exposure and response prevention in obsessive-compulsive washers. J Consult Clin Psychol 48:71–79, 1980a

Foa EB, Steketee GS, Turner RM, et al: Effects of imaginal exposure to feared disasters in obsessive-compulsive checkers. Behav Res Ther 18:449–455, 1980b

Foa EB, Grayson JB, Steketee GS: Depression, habituation and treatment outcome in obsessive-compulsives, in Learning-Theory Approaches to Psychiatry. Edited by Boulougouris J. New York, Wiley, 1982, pp 129–142

Foa EB, Steketee GS, Grayson JB, et al: Treatment of obsessive-compulsives: when do we fail? in Failures in Behavior Therapy. Edited by Foa EB, Emmelkamp PMG. New York, Wiley, 1983, pp 10–34

Foa EB, Steketee GS, Grayson JB, et al: Deliberate exposure and blocking of obsessive-compulsive rituals: immediate and long-term effects. Behavior Therapy 15:450–472, 1984

Foa EB, Steketee GS, Ozarow BJ: Behavior therapy with obsessive-compulsives: from theory to treatment, in Obsessive-Compulsive Disorder: Psychological and Pharmacological Treatment. Edited by Mavissakalian M, Turner SM, Michelson L. New York, Plenum, 1985, pp 49–129

Goodman WK, Price LH, Rasmussen SA, et al: Efficacy of fluvoxamine in obsessive-compulsive disorder: a double-blind comparison with placebo. Arch Gen Psychiatry 46:36–44, 1989a

Goodman WK, Price LH, Rasmussen SA, et al: The Yale-Brown Obsessive-Compulsive Scale (Y-BOCS), I: development, use and reliability. Arch Gen Psychiatry 46:1006–1011, 1989b

Goodman WK, McDougle CJ, Price LH, et al: Beyond the serotonin hypothesis: a role for dopamine in some forms of obsessive-compulsive disorder? J Clin Psychiatry 51:36–43, 1990a

Goodman WK, Price LH, Delgado PL, et al: Specificity of serotonin reuptake inhibitors in the treatment of obsessive-compulsive disorder: comparison of fluvoxamine and desipramine. Arch Gen Psychiatry 47:577–585, 1990b

Goodman WK, McDougle CJ, Price LH: Pharmacotherapy of obsessive-compulsive disorder. J Clin Psychiatry 53 (4, suppl):29–37, 1992

Greist JH: Treatment of obsessive-compulsive disorder: psychotherapies, drugs, and other somatic treatment. J Clin Psychiatry 51 (8, suppl):44–50, 1990

Greist JH, Chouinard G, DuBoff E, et al: Double-blind comparison of three doses of sertraline and placebo in the treatment of outpatients with obsessive-compulsive disorder. Paper presented at the 18th Collegium Internationale Neuropsychopharmacologicum Congress, Nice, France, June 29, 1992

Hodgson G, Rachman S, Marks IM: The treatment of chronic obsessive-compulsive neurosis: follow-up and further findings. Behav Res Ther 10:181–189, 1972

Hollander E: Serotonergic drugs and the treatment of disorders related to obsessive-compulsive disorder, in Current Treatments of Obsessive-Compulsive Disorder. Edited by Pato MT, Zohar J. Washington, DC, American Psychiatric Press, 1991, pp 173–191

Hollander E, Fay M, Liebowitz M: Serotonergic and noradrenergic function in obsessive-compulsive disorder. Am J Psychiatry 145:1015–1017, 1988

Hoogduin K, DeHaan E, Schaap C, et al: Exposure and response prevention in patients with obsessions. Acta Psychiatr Belg 87:640–653, 1987

Insel TR, Murphy DL, Cohen RM, et al: Clomipramine and clorgyline in OCD. Arch Gen Psychiatry 40:605–612, 1983

Jaskari MO: Observations on mianserin in the treatment of obsessive neurosis. Curr Med Res Opin 6:128–131, 1980

Jenike MA: Approaches to the patient with treatment-refractory obsessive-compulsive disorder. J Clin Psychiatry 51 (suppl):15–21, 1990a

Jenike MA: Illness related to obsessive-compulsive disorder, in Obsessive-Compulsive Disorders: Theory and Management. Edited by Jenike MA, Baer L, Minichiello WE. Chicago, IL, Year Book Medical, 1990b, pp 39–60

Jenike MA: Management of patients with treatment-resistant obsessive-compulsive disorder, in Current Treatments of Obsessive-Compulsive Disorder. Edited by Pato MT, Zohar J. Washington, DC, American Psychiatric Press, 1991, pp 135–155

Jenike MA, Hyman S, Baer L, et al: A controlled trial of fluvoxamine in obsessive-compulsive disorder: implications for a serotonergic theory. Am J Psychiatry 147:1209–1215, 1990

Jenike MA, Baer L, Buttolph L: Buspirone augmentation of fluoxetine in patients with obsessive-compulsive disorder. J Clin Psychiatry 52:12–14, 1991

Karno M, Golding JM, Sorenson SB, et al: The epidemiology of obsessive-compulsive disorder in five U.S. communities. Arch Gen Psychiatry 45:1094–1099, 1988

Kasvikis Y, Marks IM: Clomipramine in obsessive-compulsive ritualizers treated with exposure therapy: relations between dose, plasma levels, outcome and side effects. Psychopharmacology 95:113–118, 1988

Liebowitz MR, Hollander E: Obsessive-compulsive disorder: psychobiological integration, in The Psychobiology of Obsessive-Compulsive Disorder. Edited by Zohar J, Insel T, Rasmussen S. New York, Springer, 1991, pp 227–255

Marks IM: Review of behavioral psychotherapy, I: obsessive-compulsive disorders. Am J Psychiatry 138:584–592, 1981

Marks IM: Fears, Phobias and Rituals. New York, Oxford University Press, 1987

Marks IM, Stern RS, Mawson D, et al: Clomipramine and exposure for obsessive-compulsive rituals, part I. Br J Psychiatry 136:1–25, 1980

Marks IM, Lelliott P, Basoglu M, et al: Clomipramine, self-exposure and therapist-aided exposure for obsessive-compulsive rituals. Br J Psychiatry 152:522–534, 1988

Marlatt GA: Cognitive assessment and intervention procedures for relapse prevention, in Relapse Prevention: Maintenance Strategies in the Treatment of Addictive Behaviors. Edited by Marlatt GA, Gordon JR. New York, Guilford, 1985, pp 201–279

Mavissakalian MR, Jones B, Olson S: Absence of placebo response in obsessive-compulsive disorder. J Nerv Ment Dis 178:268–270, 1990

Mavissakalian MR, Turner SM, Michelson L, et al: Tricyclic antidepressants in obsessive-compulsive disorder: antiobsessional or antidepressant agents? Am J Psychiatry 142:572–576, 1985

McDougle CJ, Goodman WK, Price LH, et al: Neuroleptic addition in fluvoxamine-refractory obsessive-compulsive disorder. Am J Psychiatry 147:652–654, 1990

McDougle CJ, Goodman WK, Leckman JF, et al: Limited therapeutic effect of addition of buspirone in fluvoxamine-refractory obsessive-compulsive disorder. Am J Psychiatry 150:647–649, 1993a

McDougle CJ, Goodman WK, Leckman JF, et al: The psychopharmacology of obsessive-compulsive disorder. Psychiatr Clin North Am 16:749–766, 1993b

Meichenbaum DH: Self-instructional methods, in Helping People Change. Edited by Kanfer FH, Goldstein AF. New York, Pergamon, 1975, pp 357–392

Meichenbaum DH: Stress Inoculation Training. New York, Pergamon, 1985

Meyer V: Modification of expectations in cases with obsessional rituals. Behav Res Ther 4:273–280, 1966

Meyer V, Levy R: Modification of behavior in obsessive-compulsive disorders, in Issues and Trends in Behavior Therapy. Edited by Adams HE, Unikel P. Springfield, IL, Charles C Thomas, 1973, pp 77–137

Meyer V, Levy R, Schnurer A: A behavioral treatment of obsessive-compulsive disorders, in Obsessional States. Edited by Beech HR. London, Methuen, 1974, pp 233–258

Minichiello WE, Baer L, Jenike MA: Schizotypal personality disorder: a poor prognostic indicator for behavior therapy in the treatment of obsessive-compulsive disorder. Journal of Anxiety Disorders 1:273–276, 1987

Monteiro WO, Noshirvani HF, Marks IM, et al: Anorgasmia from clomipramine in obsessive-compulsive disorder: a controlled trial. Br J Psychiatry 151:107–112, 1987

Montgomery SA: Clomipramine in obsessional neurosis: a placebo-controlled trial. Pharmaceutical Medicine 1:189–192, 1980

Noveske FG, Hahn KR, Flynn RJ: Possible toxicity of combined fluoxetine and lithium (letter). Am J Psychiatry 146:1515, 1989

Pato MT, Zohar J: Clomipramine in the treatment of obsessive-compulsive disorder, in Current Treatments of Obsessive-Compulsive Disorder. Edited by Pato MT, Zohar J. Washington, DC, American Psychiatric Press, 1991, pp 13–28

Pato MT, Zohar-Kadouch R, Zohar J, et al: Return of symptoms after discontinuation of clomipramine in patients with obsessive-compulsive disorder. Am J Psychiatry 145:1521–1525, 1988

Perse TL, Greist JH, Jefferson JW, et al: Fluvoxamine treatment of obsessive-compulsive disorder. Am J Psychiatry 144:1543–1548, 1987

Pigott TA, Pato MT, Bernstein SE, et al: Controlled comparisons of clomipramine and fluoxetine in the treatment of OCD: behavioral and biological results. Arch Gen Psychiatry 47:926–932, 1990

Rabavilas AD, Boulougouris JC, Perissaki C: Therapist qualities related to outcome with exposure in vivo in neurotic patients. J Behav Ther Exp Psychiatry 10:293–299, 1979

Rachman S, Hodgson R: Obsessions and Compulsions. Englewood Cliffs, NJ, Prentice-Hall, 1980

Rachman S, Hodgson R, Marks IM: The treatment of chronic obsessive-compulsive neurosis. Behav Res Ther 9:237–247, 1971

Rachman S, Marks IM, Hodgson R: The treatment of obsessive-compulsive neurotics by modelling and flooding in vivo. Behav Res Ther 11:463–471, 1973

Rasmussen SA: Lithium and tryptophan augmentation in clomipramine resistant obsessive-compulsive disorder. Am J Psychiatry 141:1283–1285, 1984

Rasmussen SA, Eisen JL: Clinical features and phenomenology of obsessive-compulsive disorder. Psychiatric Annals 19:67–73, 1989

Rasmussen SA, Eisen JL: Epidemiology of obsessive-compulsive disorder. J Clin Psychiatry 51 (2, suppl):10–13, 1990

Rasmussen SA, Eisen JL: Phenomenology of OCD: Clinical subtypes, heterogeneity, and coexistence, in The Psychobiology of Obsessive-Compulsive Disorder. Edited by Zohar J, Insel T, Rasmussen S. New York, Springer, 1991, pp 13–43

Rasmussen SA, Tsuang MT: Epidemiological and clinical findings of significance to the design of neuropharmacologic studies of obsessive-compulsive disorder. Psychopharmacol Bull 22:723–733, 1986

Robins LN, Helzer JE, Weissman MM, et al: Lifetime prevalence of specific psychiatric disorders in three sites. Arch Gen Psychiatry 41:949–958, 1984

Roper G, Rachman S, Marks I: Passive and participant modelling in exposure treatment of obsessive-compulsive neurotics. Behav Res Ther 13:271–279, 1975

Salama AA, Shafey M: A case of severe lithium toxicity induced by combined fluoxetine and lithium carbonate (letter). Am J Psychiatry 146:228, 1989

Salkovskiis PM, Westbrook D: Behavior therapy and obsessional ruminations: can failure be turned into success? Behav Res Ther 27:149–169, 1989

Spiegel DA: Treatment of choice: Drugs, behavior therapy, or both? OCD Newsletter 6:1–2, 1992

Steketee GS: Personality traits and diagnoses in obsessive-compulsive disorder. Paper presented at the annual meeting of the Association for the Advancement of Behavior Therapy, New York, NY, November 1988

Steketee GS: Personality traits and disorders in obsessive-compulsives. Journal of Anxiety Disorders 4:351–364, 1990

Steketee GS: Treatment of Obsessive-Compulsive Disorder. New York, Guilford, 1993

Steketee GS, Foa EB: Obsessive-compulsive disorder, in Clinical Handbook of Psychological Disorders. Edited by Barlow DH. New York, Guilford, 1988, pp 69–143

Steketee GS, Tynes LL: Behavioral treatment of obsessive-compulsive disorder, in Current Treatments of Obsessive-Compulsive Disorder. Edited by Pato MT, Zohar J. Washington, DC, American Psychiatric Press, 1991, pp 61–86

Stern RS: Obsessive thoughts: the problem of therapy. Br J Psychiatry 133:200–205, 1978

Stern RS, Marks IM, Mawson D, et al: Clomipramine and exposure for compulsive rituals, II: plasma levels, side effects and outcome. Br J Psychiatry 136:161–166, 1980

Sternbach H: Danger of MAOI therapy after fluoxetine withdrawal (letter). Lancet 2:850–851, 1988

Swedo SE, Rapoport JL, Leonard H, et al: Obsessive-compulsive disorder in children and adolescents. Arch Gen Psychiatry 46:335–345, 1989

Telch MJ, Agras WS, Taylor CB, et al: Imipramine and behavioral treatment for agoraphobia. Behav Res Ther 13:375–383, 1985

Thorén P, Åsberg M, Cronholm B, et al: Clomipramine treatment of obsessive-compulsive disorder, I: a controlled clinical trial. Arch Gen Psychiatry 37:1281–1285, 1980

Tollefson GD, Rampey AH, Potvin JH, et al: A multicenter investigation of fixed-dose fluoxetine in the treatment of obsessive-compulsive disorder. Arch Gen Psychiatry 51:559–567, 1994

Turner SM, Jacob RG, Beidel DC, et al: Fluoxetine treatment of obsessive-compulsive disorder. J Clin Psychopharmacol 5:207–212, 1985

Van Noppen BL, Rasmussen SA, Eisen J, et al: A multifamily group approach as an adjunct to treatment of obsessive-compulsive disorder, in Current Treatments of Obsessive-Compulsive Disorder. Edited by Pato MT, Zohar J. Washington, DC, American Psychiatric Press, 1991, pp 115–134

Volavka J, Neziroglu F, Yaryura-Tobias JA: Clomipramine and imipramine in obsessive-compulsive disorder. Psychiatry Res 14:83–91, 1985

Wheadon DE: Placebo-controlled multicenter trial of fluoxetine in OCD. Paper presented at the 5th World Congress of Biological Psychiatry, Florence, Italy, June 12, 1991

Zetin M, Kramer MA: Obsessive-compulsive disorder. Hosp Community Psychiatry 43:689–699, 1992

Zohar J, Insel TR: Obsessive-compulsive disorder: psychobiological approaches to diagnosis, treatment, and pathophysiology. Biol Psychiatry 22:667–687, 1987

Zohar J, Pato MT: Diagnostic considerations, in Current Treatments of Obsessive-Compulsive Disorder. Edited by Pato MT, Zohar J. Washington, DC, American Psychiatric Press, 1991, pp 1–12

Zohar J, Mueller E, Insel T, et al: Serotonergic responsivity in obsessive-compulsive disorder: comparison of patients with healthy controls. Arch Gen Psychiatry 44:946–951, 1987

Zohar J, Zohar-Kadouch RC, Kindler S: Current concepts in the pharmacological treatment of obsessive-compulsive disorder. Drugs 43:210–218, 1992

Zohar-Kadouch R, Pato MT, Zohar J, et al: Follow-up of obsessive-compulsive patients. Paper presented at the 142nd annual meeting of the American Psychiatric Association, San Francisco, CA, May 1989

Anxiety Disorders in Children: Applying a Cognitive-Behavioral Technique That Can Be Integrated With Pharmacotherapy or Other Psychosocial Interventions

Robert G. Ziegler, M.D.

Anxiety occurs frequently in children, as it does in adults. Although anxiety symptoms can signal the presence of a more chronic anxiety disorder, they most often indicate more circumscribed reactions to environmental stresses, internal demands, or external expectations. Managing anxiety requires the development and use of coping skills, including psychological defenses, communication techniques, and problem-solving abilities. These skills are typically developed during childhood, facilitated by parental support, limit-setting behavior, and verbal exchanges that lead to the recognition of feelings and appropriate interpersonal and internal problem solving. When a child's coping skills are overwhelmed, however, overt anxiety symptoms may appear. Assessment of these symptoms involves careful examination of the child's and family's coping abilities as well as the possible contribution of a primary anxiety disorder.

Techniques that help adults to contain anxiety, such as the abilities to express feelings, accept reassurance, and test reality, also work well for children. When an adult is helping a child to cope, however, the intervention must be at the child's level of understanding. Dynamic approaches to psychotherapy (Gabbard 1992) and cognitive-behavioral approaches to anxiety disorders (see Chapter 2) have been adapted to child populations (Carlson et al. 1986; Ramirez et al. 1987).

Interventions for children with anxiety disorders have four basic components:

1. The clinician helps the child and parents understand the features of the anxiety state.
2. The clinician assists in strengthening the child's coping skills and management of anxiety.
3. Treatment helps the parents to support the child's emotional needs and to set appropriate limits on the child's behavior.
4. Treatment enhances social and emotional understanding and problem solving within the family as a whole.

Once the child's and family's abilities to identify and cope with anxiety symptoms are consolidated and they understand the importance of coping mechanisms, psychosocial communication, and problem solving, a foundation has been built for any concurrent or subsequent pharmacotherapeutic consultation. Child and parents will recognize the target symptoms, understand the diagnosis, and be ready to discuss the risks and benefits of pharmacotherapeutic interventions.

In this chapter I focus on a technique of creating books for parent and child that accomplishes all four of these objectives. Other psychodynamic and cognitive-behavioral interventions can be integrated with this technique as indicated for further management of evolving problems or symptoms. Pharmacotherapy, used in conjunction with book-making, can contribute to a child's recovery by enhancing coping skills that diminish the intensity, frequency, and impact of debilitating symptoms. In view of the paucity of data supporting pharmacotherapy as a sole treatment modality in children (Sylvester and Kruesi 1994), it is recommended that medications be prescribed within the context of a multimodal approach that integrates individual and family treatment, including parent education, drawing on the insights of dynamic and cognitive-behavioral approaches.

■ Clinical Assessment

Anxiety symptoms in a child warrant professional evaluation when those symptoms respond insufficiently to support from parents, members of the extended family, teachers, or friends. Thorough assessment of anxiety requires the clinician to gather information from all sectors of the child's life. Because much valuable data may be omitted by the child or reported only in a disguised manner, a clinician must be able to conduct a developmentally attuned play interview using both direct questioning and play exchanges. In addition, careful developmental and family histories may reveal predisposing temperamental factors within the child or levels of anxiety within the family (or environment) that are overtly or covertly communicated to the child. The history-taking can be supplemented by the use of one of the standard behavioral checklists, such as the Child Behavior Checklist (Achenbach and Edelbrock 1983) or the Conners (1969, 1973) scales, with which anxious symptomatology can be readily documented and comorbid conditions easily noted.

DSM-III-R (American Psychiatric Association 1987) defines three anxiety disorders of childhood: separation anxiety disorder (present in DSM-IV [American Psychiatric Association 1994]), overanxious disorder (*generalized anxiety disorder* in DSM-IV), and avoidant disorder (considered either *social phobia* or *avoidant per-*

sonality disorder in DSM-IV). These disorders possess features in common (see Table 7–1) and include several overlapping categories (see Figure 7–1). It is important, however, to also consider in children five other anxiety disorders defined in the adult section of DSM-III-R (change noted in DSM-IV): simple phobia *(specific phobia),* obsessive-compulsive disorder, panic disorder, posttraumatic stress disorder, and adjustment disorder with anxious mood *(with anxiety).* Agoraphobia, as defined for adult patients, usually meets the criteria for separation anxiety disorder when encountered in a child. Indeed, separation anxiety may be an important

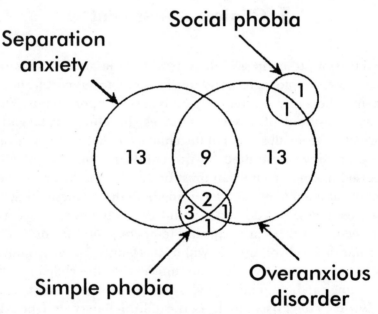

Figure 7–1. Comorbidity of anxiety disorders in a community sample of 44 adolescents and children. The numbers in the intersecting circles indicate the numbers of children and adolescents with comorbidity of the indicated disorders.

Source. Reprinted from Kashani JH, Orvaschel H: "A Community Study of Anxiety in Children and Adolescents." *American Journal of Psychiatry* 147:315, 1990. Copyright 1990, American Psychiatric Association. Used with permission.

Table 7–1.   Anxiety disorders in children (DSM-III-R)

Diagnosis	Key symptoms	Prevalence (%)
Separation anxiety disorder (Case 1)	1. Unrealistic worries about harm or loss of major figures 2. Reluctance or refusal to go to school or sleepovers 3. Complaints of physical symptoms 4. Signs of excessive distress on separating 5. Signs of poor function when separated from major attachment	3.5–6
Overanxious disorder (Case 2)	1. Unrealistic worries 2. Preoccupations with past behavior 3. Overconcern about competence 4. Excessive need for reassurance 5. Marked tension/somatization	2.7–4.6
Avoidant disorder (Case 3)	1. Persistent shrinking from contact with strangers 2. Desire/demand for acceptance from family and friends 3. Avoidant behavior with peers	Unknown
Simple phobia (Case 2)	Use adult criteria	2–50
Obsessive-compulsive disorder (Case 4)	Use adult criteria	2

(continued)

Table 7–1.   Anxiety disorders in children (DSM-III-R) *(continued)*

Diagnosis	Key symptoms	Prevalence (%)
Panic disorder (Case 1)	Use adult criteria	Unknown
Posttraumatic stress disorder	Use adult criteria	Unknown
Adjustment disorder with anxious mood (Cases 5 and 6)	Use adult criteria	Unknown

factor even in adults with panic disorder, as suggested by a recent study that showed a high prevalence of separation anxiety dreams in adults with panic disorder (Free et al. 1993).

Although comorbid disorders are not the focus of this chapter, it is important to note that anxiety disorders in children can co-occur with other psychiatric disorders such as attentional disorders, conduct disorders (Biederman et al. 1991; Plizka 1992), or mood disorders (Bernstein and Garfinkel 1986). In children who have disruptive behavior disorders, vulnerability to secondary anxiety assumes importance as they come to recognize their behavior as impulsive and to understand the risks of such behavior. At times, as with adults, it is difficult to determine whether a child's anxiety is primary or secondary to a mood disorder. A full-blown anxiety state can also represent the onset of posttraumatic stress disorder or signal a significant degree of otherwise concealed conflict within a family. The presence of any of these complicating conditions may impede a child's response to standard, multimodal treatment of anxiety, leading to a reevaluation.

■ **Case Example 1: Separation Anxiety Disorder With Depressive Symptoms**

Katie was in fourth grade when her mother brought her for psychotherapy. The mother reported that no matter how positive she was with Katie, Katie said that she was always unhappy and that nobody liked her. She seemed bored, irritable, and apathetic. Katie said she felt like she should be dead. She showed anxiety at the drop of a hat. The mother said that Katie's symptoms persisted even though the family was very proud of Katie and she had a nice circle of friends.

As the history was further explored, it became clear that Katie had shown symptoms of separation anxiety disorder since nursery school. Each morning she had tearful tantrums and clung desperately to her mother when her mother dropped her off at school. Since she had never been able to tolerate the school bus, her mother had driven her every day. Some days, as soon as they got close to the school, Katie complained of headaches and stomachaches and her mother brought her back home. Katie's mother and father fought over the mother's tendency to give in to Katie. The mother said the pediatrician had never found anything physically wrong with Katie.

Katie's separation anxiety disorder was obscured by the presence of depressive symptoms, which are present in one-third of children with separation anxiety disorder (Bernstein and Garfinkel 1986) or other forms of anxiety disorders of childhood (Francis et al. 1992). The distinction between a primary depressive disorder and depression that follows upon anxious worrying can be difficult to make at presentation. A careful history of the evolution of Katie's symptoms revealed the diagnosis. In addition, unresolved parental differences were noted that prevented the development of consistent limits in order to help Katie contain her anxiety.

■ Case Example 2: Overanxious Disorder With Comorbid Phobias, Aggression, and Attention-Deficit/Hyperactivity Disorder

Don was 8 years old when his second-grade teacher told his mother that he should have a behavioral evaluation. The teacher was most troubled by Don's aggressive behavior on the playground. The mother had already been thinking about seeking evaluation because of Don's pervasive fearfulness. Over the years, Don's mother had noted the comings and goings of various simple phobias. At some point or another, Don had reported fears of thunder, darkness, spiders, and other animals. His mother was most concerned about Don's constant worries, somatic complaints, concerns about his competence, and continual need for reassurance.

In his play interview, Don talked about how other kids didn't like him and wanted to beat him up. He had very little awareness of how his sudden angry reactions affected his playmates. His mother reported that Don's temper had been very reactive since nursery school and had continued to be so when he began public school. The abnormal Conners Scale scores obtained by both teacher and mother made apparent Don's difficulty in sustaining attention. This attentional problem was confirmed by cognitive testing with the Wechsler Intelligence Scale for Children, Third Edition (WISC-III; Wechsler 1993).

In each child evaluation, assessment includes attention to understanding the interplay between the list of problems and symptoms developed by parents and therapist, the suspected diagnostic entities, and the psychodynamics of the child and family. Careful consideration must also be given to aspects of the child's behavioral regulation that might be related to constitutional and temperamental factors; the presence of a disorder such as attention-deficit/hyperactivity disorder (ADHD), oppositional defiant disorder, or conduct disorder; and the child's attempts to comply with parental expectations. In this case, the mother's preoccupations with Don's fears drew attention away from Don's aggressive behavior and attentional difficulties.

■ Case Example 3: Avoidant Disorder With Comorbid Overanxious Disorder

Timmy, age 6, was referred for consultation following his failure to respond to a combined medical and behavioral approach to his encopresis. In the initial consultation, he sat looking wide-eyed and worried as his mother reviewed the problems he had been having with his "poops" and what the pediatrician had prescribed. When the therapist began to focus on what Timmy liked to do, Timmy refused to join the conversation, and his mother described what she had come to call his "stubbornness." With continued questioning, the mother revealed what she had accepted as Timmy's personality style: his avoidance of peers, his retreat behind her when new people arrived, and his frequent demands for reassurance.

When Timmy was seen alone, he hesitantly began to draw, and his difficulties with fine motor control were apparent. He gradually engaged with the play therapist, but only on his own very controlling terms. When this was noted to him, he quickly became anxious and made regressive play choices such as Play-Doh or games typically selected by much younger children. Timmy made lots of Play-Doh poops and once made a picture of a toilet that made him so anxious that he finally hid it under the therapist's couch. His Conners Scale scores included assessments that flagged both attentional disorder features and symptoms of an oppositional disorder. The dominant symptoms, however, indicated the presence of over-anxious disorder and avoidant disorder.

In this case, the diagnostic formulation should emphasize how this youngster's oppositional symptoms and anxiety disorders undermined the previous behavioral approach to his encopresis. At one moment he would seem too anxious to withstand limit setting, while at the next moment he would react defiantly. His developmental unevenness further contributed to his shaky self-esteem and poor compliance. Timmy's anxiety about being able to perform "as expected" diminished his ability to manage any but the most carefully designed behavioral directives.

■ Case Example 4: Obsessive-Compulsive Disorder With Depressed Mood

Eugene was referred for clinical consultation after a parent-teacher conference in second grade in which the teacher pointed out Eugene's considerable difficulties with completing his work. Most of his abilities were age-appropriate, and he had above-average language skills. He was so perfectionistic, however, that once he made an error he would not complete his work. He would scribble on his paper and sprawl across his desk, muttering, "It's too hard" or "I can't do it." He constantly sought attention and reassurance. When asked to read out loud, he said, "I can't do it because my voice doesn't have enough expression." He could not tolerate the teacher's praise because he worried he wouldn't do as well the next time, while criticism led him to repetitious negative self-statements. Recently he had begun to develop little rituals to help soothe his self-esteem following mistakes.

His parents noted that Eugene had always been easily preoccupied by his worries. When he was a preschooler, he had pulled out so much hair that he created a bald spot. When he had difficulty with something, he would subsequently avoid it. He kept his room in very careful order and became very upset when his mother moved something while cleaning. He would dwell on sad thoughts, obsess over issues of danger, and resist parental attempts to provide comfort. Eugene's parents confided that they had begun to tune him out and to experience irritation at his distress, since they felt they could not reach him.

Eugene's obsessive-compulsive disorder was complicated by depressive features, reflected by tearfulness and a focus on sad events. His trichotillomania, a variant of obsessive-compulsive disorder (Lenane et al. 1992), had simply been "tolerated" by his parents. Although Eugene actually met the full criteria for a diagnosis of obsessive-compulsive disorder, milder obsessions and compulsions can also be associated with other forms of anxiety. Clinicians should remain aware, also, that pervasive developmental disorder (Cohen et al. 1987) can be accompanied by regressive catastrophic anxiety reactions even in children who function at a higher level in other respects. Such children's resistance to change and apparently irrational insistence upon rigid routines may bring them to clinical attention during their early school years rather than sooner, because their parents may have accepted and become accustomed to their idiosyncrasies. Obsessive-compulsive disorder appears to have one of the best responses to pharmacotherapy of the childhood anxiety disorders (DeVeaugh-Geiss et al. 1992), and for this reason, medication consultation should be considered in the initial evaluation of children presenting with this problem.

Familial and Environmental Factors

The clinician must be alert in order to detect the presence of adjustment disorders that occur comorbidly with other disorders or in response to distressing life situations. Anxiety as a consequence of family violence (Kashani et al. 1992), alcoholism, or drug abuse must often be suspected. The presence of posttraumatic stress disorder, too, must be considered.

An important component of the evaluation of a child's anxiety is a direct inquiry regarding physical or sexual abuse (Helfer 1975). The somatic symptoms of anxiety must also be distinguished from those that may accompany physical illness. A child's anxiety may also represent the impact of a family member's illness on family life, which often includes increased stress and limited support. When family system and/or environmental factors play a major role in a child's anxiety, these must be identified and addressed insofar as possible.

High anxiety levels within the parents or others in a child's environment can be overtly or covertly communicated to and expressed by the child. During the diagnostic family interview, an anxious parent's disturbing communications can be detected by the therapist. Although such influence may not be the sole cause of a child's anxiety state, it can often further complicate any innate anxious predisposition and therefore must be considered in developing a treatment plan.

Biological and Temperamental Factors

Each of the three DSM-III-R childhood anxiety disorders affects 3%–5% of children (Livingston 1991), with approximately a 9% prevalence rate during a 6-month period when simple phobias, social phobias, and agoraphobia are included (Popper 1993). Beyond the organic illnesses that may present as anxiety syndromes even in children (see Chapter 8), a temperamental vulnerability may antedate the development of full-blown symptoms of anxiety. Considerable work has been done in recent years to examine the biological underpinnings that may predispose certain children to develop an anxiety disorder that may present lifelong problems.

Kagan and colleagues (1988), in a groundbreaking study, reported on reactions to novelty observed among a large series of children:

> A child's initial reaction to unfamiliar events, especially other people, is one of the few behavioral qualities that is moderately stable over time and independent of social class and intelligence test scores. About 10% to 15% of healthy 2- and 3-year-old children consistently become quiet, vigilant, and subdued in such contexts lasting from 5 to 30 minutes . . . Empirical indexes of a pair of related, but not identical, constructs in adults, often called introversion and extroversion, are among the most stable and heritable in contemporary psychology. (Kagan et al. 1988, p. 167)

According to Kagan's review of relevant animal studies, such responses are not restricted to the human species and may be correlated with demonstrable neurophysiological mechanisms. Avoidant cats, for example, have been shown to have greater neural activity in the basomedial amygdala following exposure to a rat as compared with cats that are less avoidant of novelty (Adamec and Stark-Adamec 1986). It is speculated that limbic electrophysiological activity may hold clues to a deeper understanding of the pathophysiology of anxiety.

Kagan et al. (1988) found that children who demonstrated restraint when exposed to novelty at age 2 tended to be socially avoidant and quiet even at 7 years of age when confronted by unfamiliar children or adults. Unlike Little Hans (Freud 1909/1955), who had a simple phobia (Spitzer et al. 1981), some inhibited children may experience a generalization of phobia to other stimuli. Little Hans had a phobia restricted to horses, which led Freud to speculate about the phobia's association with the boy's concurrent interest in his "widdler." In children with overanxious disorder, however, a simple phobic reaction to horses could conceivably spread to other animals and then even to a wide range of hairy or furry objects (Jones 1924; Watson and Rayner 1920). Secondary anticipatory anxiety—prompted by the thought of encounters with these objects—can promote generalized avoidance of places where the child anticipates having such encounters, not unlike the adult patient's secondary avoidance following the onset of panic disorder (National Institute of Mental Health 1993). A vicious cycle composed of easily aroused anxiety reactions and the child's subsequent internal discomfort and avoidance may impair the possibility for developing better means of coping with stressful stimuli.

Because the parents of children with a predisposition to withdraw from novelty are themselves likely to have anxiety difficulties, the possibility exists that such parents unintentionally reinforce the child's anxious responses. When an anxious parent is too easily aroused and overly empathizes with the child's distress, an intrafamilial maladaptive pattern can be consolidated that enhances the child's withdrawal tendency. As a result, the child's ability to generate better coping skills through familiar support in tolerating exposure to the feared stimulus is impaired (Livingston 1991). The helpful or harmful impact of the match between a parent's response and a child's temperamental predisposition (Thomas and Chess 1977; Turecki and Tonner 1985) can be assessed by the therapist and provides an important area for intervention.

Follow-up research on the children studied by Kagan and colleagues (Biederman et al. 1990, 1993b) has emphasized the higher risk of behaviorally inhibited children for developing anxiety disorders. Higher rates of both avoidant disorder and separation anxiety disorder developed in these children. In addition, 75% of the children with separation anxiety later developed agoraphobia. In contrast, only 7% of children without earlier behavioral inhibition and separation anxiety disorder later developed agoraphobia. Furthermore, Rosenbaum et al. (1992) reported that, compared with parents of noninhibited children, parents of inhibited children with an anxiety disorder were themselves more likely to meet criteria for diagnosis of two or more anxiety disorders. In addition to these possibly genetic factors, children of anxious parents are exposed to environmental effects that may increase the likelihood of developing an anxiety disorder. These effects include "insecure attachment" (Manassis et al. 1994), behavioral inhibition, and an excessively controlled environment (Messer and Beidel 1994).

The central nervous system (CNS) underpinnings of the predisposition to anxious response deserve attention because they provide suggestions for psychopharmacological research and treatment. Both the benzodiazepines and the tricyclic antidepressants (TCAs), currently the two most carefully researched and frequently prescribed classes of medication for anxiety disorders in children (Popper 1993), affect CNS mechanisms that influence anxiety. Future medication research, including investigation of the role of selective serotonin reuptake inhibitors (SSRIs), will continue to target more and more selectively some of those centers of the brain that are related to affective modulation and anxiety control.

Kagan and colleagues' (1988) research suggests to the clinician that the temperamental predispositions of children require appropriate supports within their developmental context to help them develop coping techniques. In addition, the persistence of anxiety symptoms (see Figure 7–2) makes a longer-term adaptive orientation in therapeutic work with children and their families valuable as a means of enhancing the patients' capacities for adapting to future stresses (Verhulst and van der Ende 1992). In addition, given the limited availability of data regarding long-term effects of pharmacotherapy on brain and other bodily tissues, pharmacotherapy is generally to be avoided as a sole first approach to the treatment of anxiety in a child. In Popper's (1993) words, "clinicians may find it a challenge to disclose full and appropriate information to parents who give informed consent for these treatments" (p. 53). As a result, psychotherapeutic work must be directed first toward developing coping skills in the child that can be supported by the family and then toward understanding how to identify a reappearance of symptoms that may require further treatment.

Cognitive and Developmental Issues

In addition to the issues of temperament in childhood, clinicians must consider the role of cognitive capacities, such as the ability to generate hypotheses about the future and to categorize and assimilate experiences. Because such (cognitive) capacities are limited in children, a child can be more easily overwhelmed. Throughout the preschool era and early childhood, the rate of phobic reactions among children can approach 50% (Popper 1993). Coming to understand the world creates some risks. For example, when a 2-year-old made the connection between teeth and biting (stated as a hypothesis: if an animal has teeth, then it can bite), farm creatures that had previously been a source of delight became objects of a phobic preoccupation, repetitively discussed as a "horsie bite." The child began to avoid not only animals but even their pictures. Another young

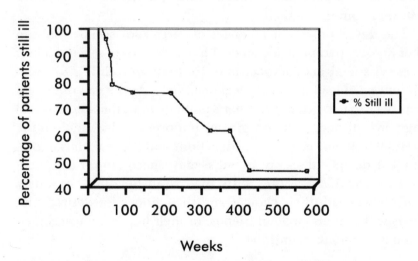

Figure 7–2. Time to recovery: anxiety disorders (*N*= 38).
Source. Reprinted from Keller MB, Lavori P, Wunder J, et al: "Chronic Course of Anxiety Disorders in Children and Adolescents." *Journal of the American Academy of Child and Adolescent Psychiatry* 31:597, 1992. Copyright 1992, American Psychiatric Association. Used with permission.

child, upon developing the capacity to classify things as "good" or "bad," became so anxiously preoccupied about the goodness or badness of his own behavior that he would on occasion be unable to choose what to do.

A child's capacity to create hypotheses and categories that shape coping responses or phobic avoidance (Gorman et al. 1989) is part of the continuing interrelatedness of inner experience with experience of the environment. The associations of emotions with hypotheses and categorizations can be sources of much anxiety during the preschool era and can complicate both the child's and the parents' lives. Helping children to use and correct the misconceptions created by their immature cognitive abilities requires the ability to patiently and repeatedly review each child's concerns. In contrast, one can imagine the complications posed for a child whose parent either is phobic of animals or responds rigidly and punitively to "good" and "bad" behaviors. The child's cognitive development occurs in a family context that can either ameliorate and create new pathways of management for all of these reactions or further complicate them.

The developmental challenges of early adolescence usher in other preoccupations associated with perceptions of self and other; identity, social acceptance, and conflicts pertaining to independence can lead to a great deal of anxiety. As the preadolescent gains the capacity to take another's point of view, the opinions and judgments of peers take on greater importance. In addition, the potential link between one's own actions and the reactions of others ("If I do this, then my friend(s) may choose to do that") becomes clearer. Preadolescents may then become anxiously preoccupied with their choices and their hopes for desired outcomes within their circle of friends, or their hopes to be accepted by a new group (Cotton 1994).

Psychodynamic Factors

Just as children's cognitive capacities affect their ability to withstand anxiety, so, too, do their psychodynamics enhance or impair their efforts to resolve ambivalent feelings, process their experiences, and understand internal conflicts generated by reality challenges to their wishes and longings. In many instances, child therapists will see anxious children whose compliant, worried demeanors conceal underlying aggressive needs or competitive drives. In other cases, the conflict between regressive wishes and independent strivings produces an inhibited and anxious veneer. Issues associated with reactions to prior loss that have become internalized and unconscious may trigger anxiety reactions within the context of a child's relationships to peers or adults. For some children, the desire for total control becomes associated with a dread of losing control that is then projected onto the world, making it a frightening place. Anxiety reactions based on these and other internal conflicts can be accessed through play therapy techniques (Schaefer 1976), Draw-a-Person tests and kinetic family drawings (e.g., Di Leo 1973), sentence completion tests, and other forms of psychological testing.

▌ Treatment Planning

The DSM-III-R anxiety disorders of childhood respond well to a combination of treatment techniques. An integrated approach may include guidance of parental behavior, cognitive-behavioral interventions, free-play interviews, and directed family interviews that strengthen family communication and coping skills. Pharmacotherapy, when appropriate, can provide additional benefit. When the child has parents that can respond constructively to the therapist's suggestions about how to reassure the child *and* how to limit the child's negative behavioral reactions, the prognosis is improved (Livingston 1991).

A model I have found useful in treating anxiety disorders includes four tasks. This model draws upon a previous view of task-focused treatment for children and families (Ziegler 1980).

Task 1. *Instruct both child and parent about the nature and symptomatology of the anxiety disorders.* Understanding anxiety symptoms, their triggers, and their courses is important, given that such symptoms tend to recur and remit throughout the life course. The clinician must also explain to parents and child the importance of influential emotional triggers, because the therapist's psychodynamic understanding (Shear et al. 1993) can aid in treatment planning. Other mood or behavioral disturbances that coexist with the anxiety disorder should be identified and explained in ways that ease parental acceptance of the child's difficulties. At the same time, clearly elucidating the symptoms, their triggers, and how parent and child can understand these will enable the therapist to help the child comprehend the focus and process of therapy.

Task 2.   *Strengthen the child's coping skills and ability to manage anxiety.*

Task 3.   *Facilitate parental support of the child's emotional needs and social development while setting appropriate limits on behaviors that undermine self-esteem and family comfort.* Although familial and extrafamilial supports are important in all of the anxiety reactions of childhood, the value of appropriate limits should also be recognized. In the terminology of the behavioral school, limits function in the service of desensitization. They say to the child, "Even frightening experiences can be tolerated if addressed repetitively in tolerable amounts." Families that fail to set limits may enhance a child's vulnerability to anxiety, fostering the development of multiple fears and tyrannical behavior (Livingston 1991). An aspect of this task that often presents both difficulties and rewards is the process of helping parents to identify and alter behaviors of their own that contribute to the child's difficulties. Parental mental disorders, in this context, should be identified and treated.

Task 4.   *Ensure that the psychotherapeutic techniques lay the groundwork for the child's constructive future development.* The therapy should enhance the child's ability to communicate with the family about social and emotional issues in order to promote productive problem solving about these issues.

Many different techniques can be used to reach these four objectives. Free-play sessions can access unconscious reactions to stresses and help the child experience relief from the worry that certain emotions are unacceptable. This can diminish the child's defensive reactions and increase his or her acceptance of the reassurance and direction that the parents have learned to offer under therapeutic guidance. During the course of the treatment, family members should develop a better understanding of anxiety, of how the child feels, and of how those feelings affect the child's behavior within the family unit.

In this era of managed care, techniques that help to define a circumscribed problem and to focus interventions are increasingly sought. The more dynamically oriented clinician will find that using a focused technique with anxious children is, paradoxically, quite liberating for both the child and the family because it helps them channel their efforts effectively. In addition, since anxiety often prompts emotional constriction and defensiveness, once the child and family are focused on working together with the therapist to diminish these very troubling feelings, they will be more able to handle explorations of the anger and sadness that often exacerbate or complicate anxiety symptoms.

Pharmacotherapeutic interventions may play a supplementary role when anxious symptomatology is not contained with psychotherapy alone. The primary therapist, using the book-making technique described in the following section, can facilitate the integration of pharmacotherapy by preparing a clear symptom list that can provide useful data for the consulting pharmacotherapist. By communicating genuine respect for the child's suffering and making use of the child's and family's strengths in the psychotherapeutic treatment, the therapist will also help clear the way for all concerned to accept consideration of whether medications can play a role as another "helper." The most urgent indications for medication use occur with children suffering from separation anxiety disorder, obsessive-compulsive disorder, or panic disorder. Medications may diminish the intensity of these syndromes' symptoms and allow other aspects of the child's treatment to be further defined and structured.

A pharmacotherapy consultation may be insisted upon by

those families that have a highly medicalized view of treatment. Such parents may need the "medication consultant" to validate the importance of solving problems, building coping skills, and communicating within the family. If the psychotherapist uses the technique described in this chapter, the consulting pharmacotherapist's role will emerge readily. The collaborative nature of the goal of enhancing the child's functioning will be clear to the consultant, as will the identified target symptoms.

As is discussed later in this chapter, the specific pharmacotherapeutic interventions for children with anxiety disorders must work hand in hand with the designated behavioral and dynamically attuned individual and family treatment.

▌ Book Making: A Technique for Focusing Treatment With Anxious Children and Families

One way to lay the groundwork for each of the four major components of the treatment plan for anxious children and their families (Ziegler 1992) is to create books for, and with, children. The purpose of such books is to enhance the child's ability to

▌ Identify and understand his or her feelings (and symptoms)
▌ Understand his or her situation better, including the psychosocial triggers of anxiety as well as possible internal conflicts that promote anxiety
▌ Define and strengthen the coping techniques that will be reinforced and supported by the parents, including enhanced communication and problem solving about psychosocial issues

A book written by a child in collaboration with a psychotherapist or parent provides a natural vehicle both for achieving an understanding of the child's problems and for identifying possible interventions. In certain instances, making a book for a child (and, indirectly, for the parents) will also clarify the context and development of the child's difficulty. Thereafter, subsequent books can define and reinforce the coping techniques suggested by the therapist. Each book should be designed to describe the child's feelings or the situation in a low-key, nonjudgmental way and should set the stage for the new steps of a behavioral program, a relaxation exercise, or a problem-solving technique. By making a story, the therapist can create an affectively neutral cognitive perspective. Children can use the assistance of therapist-made books to deal with their experiences, including the ones that have brought them into treatment.

Children often need an adult's help in constructing a complete picture. They cannot easily integrate the elements of "the story" or all of the feelings they are experiencing. The overview provided by the therapeutic understanding in the book is enhanced by the patience and concern the parent manifests in reading the book with the child. Describing a situation can be the first objective of a therapeutic book. Children's feelings are a big part of what they experience. Because such feelings are intense and often lead to immediate reactions, children need help in identifying and accepting them. A therapeutic book can help both parents and child to tolerate these feelings by describing the child's behavior in a nonjudgmental way. Thus, as children read about a situation and their reactions, the stage is set for them to "discover" and label their feelings.

Labeling feelings may be more natural for some families than for others. When a therapist creates a story, the way the story is framed can diminish the parent's reactivity as well as the child's. The child may respond to a situation with both behavior and feelings that may appear to the parent as irritability, lack of cooperation, unwanted fretfulness, or stubbornness. Acceptance is the way to help children identify and understand their feelings. Of course, children can test the limits of a parent's ability to admit, accept, and describe behavior. The therapist must take an active hand in this process of understanding. Acceptance can be modeled in the book made for the symptomatic child by adding a general closing statement that expresses empathy for the child.

■ **Case Example 5: Adjustment
Disorder With Anxious Mood**

One family came for consultation following their 8-year-old
son's loss of previously attained coping skills. Billy had begun
having trouble leaving home to go to the school bus stop. He
showed increased stubbornness about completing the tasks assigned to him at home and school, and he manifested a general
sense of gloom, anxiety, and irritability. The parents were
quite certain that these reactions had developed following the
mother's return to work and her new unavailability for one of
the week nights. There was also an increased pace and sense
of pressure within the family.

The consultant recommended making a book to help Billy
with his feelings; however, because the parent's direct inquir-
ies about the boy's feelings had been unfruitful, an indirect
tactic was adopted in making the book. Instead of focusing on
Billy's feelings, the book was directed toward the details of the
new family routines to help Billy see the new situation more
clearly and to accept his own reactions.

This was the book that Billy's parents were able to make
during the consultation:

■ *The Family's Week*

Page 1.   Sunday is a day that our family is together. We
plan a lot of different things to do.

Page 2.   Monday, Mom brings Billy and Adam back to
school. Dad goes to work and picks up kids after school.
Mom comes home from work for supper.

Page 3.   Tuesday is a new kind of day. Mom drops kids
off at school, but she isn't home for supper. She has a new
job. Dad makes supper with Billy and Adam. We eat supper without Mom.

Page 4.   Wednesday both Billy and Adam go to karate after school. Mom brings them there and brings
them home. Wednesday is Daddy's late night at

work so we have a snack after karate before we eat supper with Dad.

Page 5. Thursday and Friday are kind of the same.
Work for Mom and Dad and school for the kids.

Page 6. Saturday is a busy day for everyone. Sometimes there are soccer games and sometimes we all go to
the playground.

After the family read the book together for 2 nights, Billy
went off to draw in his bedroom with crayons and paper. He
said he wanted to make a new cover for their book. He came
back with a new cover that said

I Hate Toosday

Billy's "I Hate Toosday" cover did two things. It clarified
what he was mad and sad about. It also showed how the family's book had helped him to organize his experience so that
he could share his feelings in a more specific way. Once that
was accomplished, Billy became more comfortable and cooperative with the new routines.

For anxious children, situations and feelings are often inter-
twined. Sometimes the therapeutic intervention can focus on the
situation and clarify the feelings; at other times, understanding and
describing the feelings helps the child understand the situation.

A book designed by the therapist in collaboration with the parents can help a child gain and keep a sense of perspective. This
new prespective can be reinforced by adding a general statement
or conclusion. For instance, a page could be added to the book for
Billy, after he had made his cover, that said, "Sometimes there are
days that are really tough for everybody," and then the whole family could make a page about the day of the week they hate most to
reinforce the sense that "there are these days, one has to cope, and
we're all in this together."

Here, in summary, are three techniques to use in the initial books that can be written for children within the treatment context. These techniques can help the therapist identify anxiety reactions and lay the groundwork to begin to establish new coping skills in the follow-up books.

1. Describe the situation nonjudgmentally.
2. Describe the child's behavior as a way to begin to label the feelings.
3. Make a general and empathic statement using "sometimes" to foster the child's acceptance of his or her situation and feelings.

Applying the Book-Making Technique to the Treatment of Anxiety Disorders

Problems with separation anxiety may become manifest when youngsters are placed in day care, when they begin kindergarten, or even during later school years. In addition, moves or changes in family life, especially for an anxious child, may precipitate more clingy or tearful behavior, irritability or stubbornness, and a heightened reactivity to situations that previously were managed well. In such situations, making a book that describes the change and its components can help. The book can list the details of the day, the nature of leave-taking, and the routine for being picked up as the basis for the therapeutic intervention. In addition, the story can focus on managing both the child's and the parent's behavior: the therapist's description of the new routine can specify rewards for the child's behavior and—in situations in which the parent has become part of the cycle of reactivity—the new behavior required from the parent. In clarifying how "Mommy will say goodbye," for example, the story can reinforce parental limit setting and create a new climate of predictability. Even when there is continued tearfulness, the child can earn a star for saying goodbye. Limits that foster predictability, understanding of the difficult moment, and acceptance of the feelings are the cornerstone of this cognitive-behavioral intervention that can address the feelings and behavior of both the anxious child and the family. In many cases of this kind, the full-blown picture of a separation anxiety disorder may not be present.

■ Case Example 6: Adjustment Disorder With Anxious Mood (and Separation Anxiety)

Talisha, a 3-year-old with an anxious temperament, responded to starting day care with tearfulness, difficulty separating, and tantrums when being picked up after day care. To help contain the child's difficulties and her mother's reactivity, the therapist helped the two to create a storybook called *My New School,* combined with a series of stars for "no more tantrums" that led to a special game-playing time for mother and child. Also included in the intervention was a calendar that had "purple days" (Talisha's favorite color) for school days so that the little girl could check the calendar herself to see whether she needed to go to day care on a specific day. The therapist, who remained in intermittent long-term contact with this family, subsequently learned that at each new school-year transition, Talisha would ask for her *My New School* book to help her adjust to saying goodbye again. Talisha continued this request until entering third grade, when she decided it was time to put her book in her memory box.

In this example, a parent's ability to offer structured information in a supportive way helped her child to adjust to a series of difficult transitions. In the process, the child consolidated a new set of coping skills and accepted the limit that she had to say goodbye and go to school. In treatment of the full panoply of symptoms of separation anxiety disorder (as in Case Example 1), the skills of the psychotherapist are needed to direct and guide parental behavior as well as to assess the child's reactions.

■ Treatment of Case Example 1 (Separation Anxiety Disorder With Depressive Features)

Although Katie's book was intended to help her understand her feelings, it also had to reinforce the limit that even though "sometimes kids feel bad when they start off their day at school, it's a job that has to be done." To facilitate the new routine, the therapist suggested that Katie's father be the person to drop off Katie, and her mother would pick her up. A new behavioral program was also structured to reward Katie for these transitions and to work toward having Katie use the bus with her friends. As Katie accomplished the goals spelled out in each "new edition" of her books, she began to feel better about herself, assume more independence, and experience more security in her friendships.

Two years later, however, Katie developed the symptoms of a panic disorder. Previously, medication had been suggested during the initial difficult move toward the school bus, but her parents felt that adhering to the limits defined in her therapy permitted Katie's best adjustment and reasonable coping. At this point, however, Katie's symptoms were severe enough—and she could recognize them clearly as a result of her prior treatment—to warrant referral for pharmacotherapy. The therapist recommended that Katie and her parents make a list of Katie's experiences and the parents' new observations.

This next phase of treatment allowed Katie to meet with a psychiatrist in order to describe her symptoms with her parents' support. She was offered a trial of an antidepressant, which successfully alleviated her panic symptoms.

In children who present with anxiety, the treating clinician must be alert for signs of the onset of panic disorder before or during adolescence, because this occurs frequently (see Figure 7–3). Pharmacotherapy is an important consideration in the treatment of these youngsters. Although large-scale, controlled studies of children with panic disorder are still lacking and those available are confounded by the high rate of placebo responses among children and adolescents (Popper 1993), many anecdotal reports have described positive results from pharmacotherapeutic intervention (Joorabchi 1977; Kutcher and MacKenzie 1988; Steingard 1993), although consistent confirmation is lacking (Bernstein et al. 1990).

Instead of a book-making technique, teenagers with anxiety problems can benefit from using a paper-and-pencil listing technique in which their symptoms can be reviewed and defined. The cognitive-behavioral strategies helpful with adults (Barlow 1992; Burns 1990) can be adapted for children to help them move from listing feelings to clarifying what they think about when these feelings occur, and finally to make "thought corrections" that may result in better coping techniques.

■   **Treatment of Case Example 2
(Overanxious Disorder With Comorbid
Phobias, Aggression, and ADHD)**

Don's treatment book was focused on helping Don notice his angry feelings. The first book was presented as a "detective story" in which Don had to gather information about the situations in which he was asked to "stop and think" about his

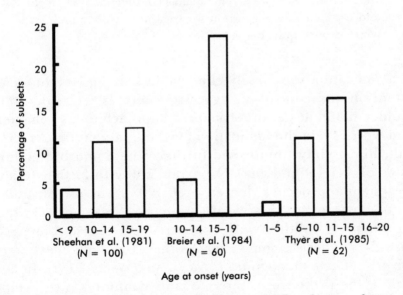

Figure 7–3.   Retrospective reports of age at childhood onset of panic. *Source.*   Reprinted with permission from Moreau D, Weissman M: "Panic Disorder in Children and Adolescents: A Review." *American Journal of Psychiatry* 149:1307, 1992. Copyright 1992, American Psychiatric Association. Used with permission.

behavior. This was a phrase that the therapist asked both family members and school personnel to employ in helping Don to complete his first book of "times when bad things happened." Another book was also started, called *My Worry Book,* to help Don notice when he was anxious. Following these explorations, appropriate limits were incorporated into star charts to help Don feel proud about "bossing my mad feelings" and "being brave with my worried feelings." This intervention increased Don's peer awareness and diminished some of his anxiety.

Although the behavioral program enhanced Don's self-control, he continued to be quite impulsive. Once the comorbid problem of an attentional disorder was identified and addressed, the parents were able to accept the importance of collaborating with a medication consultation. At this point, both Don and his parents knew how the therapist's techniques were helping and what they wanted to discuss as target symptoms with the doctor. Pharmacotherapeutic consultation was sought and resulted in a suggestion for treatment with stimulants, which proved quite helpful.

Medication was clearly effective in helping Don to focus attention and control his aggressive impulses (Ziegler and Holder 1988), just as the structured approach to his behavior and worries laid the foundation for the intervention. As a result, his anxiety diminished further. The comorbid conditions of ADHD and anxiety warrant study to further refine treatment approaches (Jensen et al. 1993). The use of stimulants, however, is an area of continuing controversy in the treatment of children with concurrent ADHD and anxiety disorders. There is some concern that stimulants may exert adverse effects on cognition (Aman and Werry 1982). In addition, the presence of internalizing symptoms (i.e., symptoms of anxiety or depression) may indicate a lesser likelihood of response to methylphenidate (DuPaul et al. 1994). TCAs remain a frequent recommendation for pharmacotherapy when ADHD is associated with significant anxiety (Ambrosini et al. 1993).

■ **Treatment of Case Example 3 (Avoidant Disorder
    With Comorbid Overanxious Disorder)**

The intensity of Timmy's anxiety and his tendency to regress led
the psychotherapist to give Timmy a number of unstructured
play sessions to enhance his comfort, facilitate his alliance with
the therapist, and prepare him for a new attempt at the behavioral
program. The play therapy required associated parent meetings
to reassure the parents—who were quite focused on getting
Timmy trained—that the free-play sessions were designed to prepare Timmy to notice his smelly pants problem and to realize
that he'd like to overcome it. At the same time, the parents
needed reminding that Timmy was quite anxious, regressed easily, and would ignore any training program that he felt he
couldn't do or for which he felt he did not have enough family
support. The parents were also going to have to monitor and
remind Timmy of the early steps of the program. After Timmy's
considerable anxiety had lessened and the parents were prepared, a book was written with Timmy to explain "the trouble I
have with my poops." Timmy was given a simple calendar in
which to note "BM days" and "P" days (when he lost control of
his urine). The calendar, and his faithful cooperation in keeping
it, set the stage to begin a program that combined medications
and acceptable toilet-sitting times. Timmy really wanted to help
himself "be a big boy the way he'd like to be." He was ready to
face the toilet! In this case, the collaboration with Timmy's pediatrician was reinforced.

Desensitization—the graduated exposure of the child to one
or more feared objects—is an active program for increasing self-
control. It is typically combined with relaxation training. Goldfried (1971) defines desensitization as a cognitively mediated
process that behaviorists advocate as one approach to coping
with anxiety. Therapeutic books can outline the steps of the exposure to the concern-provoking situations. To facilitate the
process of identifying and understanding the effects of tension,
special modifications in the relaxation program may be needed
for children. One such behavioral script is illustrated by Koep-

pen (1974) as way to help a child control tension in the neck and associated muscle groups:

> Now pretend you are a turtle. You're sitting out on a rock by a nice, peaceful pond, just relaxing in the warm sun. It feels nice and warm. Oh-oh! You sense danger. Pull your head into your house. Try to pull your shoulders up to your ears and push your head down into your shoulders. Hold in tight. It isn't easy to be a turtle in a shell. The danger is past now. You can come out into the warm sunshine. . . . Okay, you can relax now. Bring your head out and let your shoulders relax. . . . (repeated several times) . . . Notice how much better it feels to be relaxed than to be all tight. . . . There's no more danger. Nothing to worry about. Nothing to be afraid of. You feel good. (Koeppen 1974, p. 524)

Similar exercises can be incorporated into books and/or tapes to help the child and parents practice at home. A variety of cognitive-behavioral techniques have been adapted for use with children. Once the child and parents are appropriately prepared, these anxiety-reduction measures can become another focus in the treatment. Table 7–2 lists many of the approaches that can be used to manage anxiety or to change behavioral responses in children.

Applying the Book-Making Technique to the Treatment of Adjustment Disorders With Anxious Symptoms

Anxiety Associated With Medical Illnesses

Behavioral relaxation training (Carlson et al. 1986) and behavioral methods (Gilham 1990) have been used with children who experience anxiety in association with seizure disorders. Psychoeducation, too, can help both child and parents to reduce the anxieties associated with this disorder (Jan et al. 1991; Ziegler 1981). Other childhood medical disorders deserve a similar approach to help contain anxiety and enhance collaboration with medical treatment. Anxiety, for example, may be a significant component of certain neurological movement disorders such as Tourette's syndrome, Sydenham's chorea, or post–infectious encephalitis (Swedo and Leonard 1994). The parents who are most able to apply these approaches without psychotherapeutic support tend to be college educated and middle income. Research

---

Table 7–2.   Some cognitive-behavioral techniques for anxiety management

---

1. **Relaxation training**—Teaches a child methods for self-calming and self-control that can be useful in managing uncomfortable affects, including anxiety.

2. **Systematic desensitization**—Helps inhibit the anxiety response by teaching the child to reduce anxiety—for example, through relaxation training—and, through practice, to gradually increase skill in maintaining the relaxed state in the face of exposure to anxiety-inducing triggers.

3. **Cognitive procedures**—Help the child learn positive statements about the self (e.g., "I'm brave") or the situation (e.g., "snakes are funny animals"); or provide mental statements refocusing the child's mind away from anxiety-eliciting self-statements (e.g., "I feel really frightened" to a pleasant rhyme or tune.

4. **Flooding or implosive therapy**—Exposes the child to a highly anxiety-provoking stimulus until the anxiety response is extinguished; can be done in imagination.

5. **Modeling**—Shows the child examples of someone coping with a noxious stimulus or situation (e.g., showing a child films of children being prepared for a surgical procedure).

6. **Reinforced practice**—Gradually helps the child cope with a step-by-step exposure to the stimulus, with mastery at each step encouraged and supported.

7. **Exposure**—Involves introducing the child to a feared stimulus in imagination or in vivo.

8. **Response prevention**—Involves blocking the child's anxious or obsessive response to the anxiety-inducing or ritual-producing stimulus. In the treatment of obsessive-compulsive disorder in children, exposure is linked with psychoeducation and response prevention (March et al. 1994; see also Chapter 6 of this book).

into the mother-child relationship in epilepsy has also indicated the importance of the parents' ability to use educational supports to enhance their child's adaptation, especially when the parents can support task completion, offer emotional support, and enhance the child's ability to be self-reliant (Lothman and Pianta 1993).

Research on children with leukemia has stressed that the adequate functioning of these children and their families is associated with the use of healthy coping strategies such as "problem solving, a positive outlook, and good communication" (Brown et al. 1992, p. 495). Although the therapeutic intervention may focus on the child's needs, the intervention must also incorporate the family's skills to ensure the best possible long-term outcome. A skilled therapist can write a book that supports the child while offering guidance and reassurance to the family.

Psychotherapeutic books are not just for younger children with anxiety about an illness. Older school-age children can actually participate at a deeper level in the process of defining and implementing the production of a book. They can more independently follow up themes that are defined by the therapist as well as illustrate their own books. For children with chronic illnesses, a book can provide a base for use in the classroom as a science project. The fundamental technique, in which the therapist authors or jointly with a parent or parents coauthors the text, can be adapted according the child's resources. Duotherapy (Lyman and Selman 1985), involving work with two children at the same time, has been used to help children work on their individual and peer problems. It can make use of the book-making technique described here and be applied to children who are struggling to understand the impact of a medical illness. Two 11-year-old girls, for example, worked together in therapy on a book entitled *It's a Drag to Be Sick*. One girl was in treatment for juvenile diabetes and the other for scoliosis and epilepsy.

Adjustment Disorders With Anxious Mood Following Familial Stresses

For some children, anxiety and fear are part of their response to general familial stresses, such as a divorce, the loss of a cherished grandparent, or a temporary family conflict. For other children, day-to-day experience brings trauma because of the unpredictable, angry, or violent behavior of family members. For these children, there is a double jeopardy. First, a high incidence of parental anxiety or depression, alcoholism, or major mental illness has been reported in families in which violence occurs (Kashani et al. 1992). Second, these children may manifest anxiety as part of a generalized posttraumatic stress disorder (AACAP 1988; Kiser et al. 1991) and may gradually need to learn to differentiate their fear and diffuse anxiety from anger and disappointment (Lewis 1992).

■ **Case Example 7: Adjustment Disorder With Anxious Mood and "Performance Anxiety"**

Charlie was brought to therapy as a condition for returning to his regular classroom; otherwise, the family was told, he would need to be placed in a substantially separate classroom. The teacher observed a great deal of performance anxiety inhibiting the work of a talented youngster who quickly destroyed projects that showed signs of imperfection. When his mother brought Charlie into the room, she looked overtired and anxious. She immediately reported that her husband could not come because he was on the verge of losing his maintenance job and had to have 100% attendance there. Charlie appeared anxious throughout the discussion and said little. His individual play interviews, his Draw-a-Person test, and his kinetic family drawing were unrevealing. He gravitated toward structured games or played with army men, who joined opposing teams that wiped each other out, leaving a lone survivor.

Charlie's behavioral difficulties in the classroom led his mother to feel overwhelmed and confused. She just "wanted the school to handle it." Gradually, an alliance was developed with the mother by including time with Charlie, conjoint time with his mother, and sessions with Mom alone during each weekly meeting. Eventually, Charlie's mother, using the structure of the behavioral charts made during therapy with Charlie, became able to reward him appropriately for self-control.

During one exercise, in which Charlie had to put a nickel of his allowance in a "swear jar" every time he cursed, it was revealed that other family members also cursed. The mother was able to get the whole family to join in this intervention and, at the end of the week, whoever had put in the fewest nickels got to decide how the money would be spent—on an activity the family could do together.

By the ninth month of therapy, Charlie was functioning better in the classroom and his mother reported that her husband had discussed coming to a family meeting. In Charlie's play interview, he revealed that Dad had taken the money from the swear jar and had gone out to drink. Charlie said he was willing to discuss this problem with his mother, so she joined him in the session, and her husband's pattern of episodic alcohol abuse was revealed. At this point, Charlie's pervasive anxiety associated with his conflicts about anger, self-assertion, and concerns about the future became more understandable.

With his mother's help, Charlie made a book about the bad times and the good times in the family that revealed the impact of his father's episodic drinking. After much preparation, both Charlie and his mother were ready to show this book to the father and invite him to a family meeting to discuss it. To their surprise, Charlie's father was receptive, and a new stage of treatment was begun.

▌ Pharmacotherapy Referrals

The pharmacotherapy of children with anxiety disorders is a frontier characterized by excitement and hope, as increasing data are gathered. Numerous studies and ample case experiences already serve to offer preliminary guidelines for referral and treatment of a number of disorders. Table 7–3 presents a list of medications used for the most thoroughly studied childhood anxiety disorders. In view of the limited and sometimes inconsistent published results available, pharmacotherapy is not considered the sole or the first choice for many children with anxiety disorders.

The most firmly established pharmacotherapeutic approaches to child and adolescent anxiety disorders are those for the treatment of separation anxiety disorder (school phobia), panic disor-

Table 7–3.   Medications used in children with anxiety disorders

Diagnosis	Medications	Typical side effects
Overanxious disorder	Benzodiazepines (clonazepam, alprazolam)	Drowsiness, disinhibition, agitation, confusion, depression
	Azapirones (buspirone)	Nausea, headache
	Antihistamines (diphenhydramine, hydroxyzine)	Sedation, anticholinergic effects
Avoidant disorder	Benzodiazepines	As above
	SSRIs (fluoxetine, sertraline)	Irritability, insomnia, headache, nausea, diarrhea, anxiety, tremor
	Beta-blockers (propranolol)	Nausea, sedation
	TCAs (imipramine, amitriptyline)	Dry mouth, constipation, blurred vision, hypotension, sedation, weight change, electrocardiogram changes
	MAOIs (phenelzine)	Hypotension, dietary restrictions
Separation anxiety disorder (school refusal)	TCAs	As above
	Benzodiazepines	As above
Panic disorder	TCAs	As above
	Benzodiazepines	As above
Obsessive-compulsive disorder	TCA (clomipramine)	As above
	Benzodiazepines	As above
	SSRIs	As above
Posttraumatic stress disorder	Beta-blockers	As above
	Alpha$_2$-blockers (clonidine)	Sedation, hypotension, dry mouth, confusion, depression

Note.   MAOI = monoamine oxidase inhibitor; SSRI = selective serotonin reuptake inhibitor; TCA = tricyclic antidepressant.
Source.   Adapted from Biederman 1991 and Popper 1993.

der, obsessive-compulsive disorder, and attentional disorders with comorbid anxiety or depression. In addition, a report on the treatment of elective mutism with fluoxetine (Black and Uhde 1994) has encouraged hope regarding treatment of avoidant disorder of childhood (replaced in DSM-IV with social phobia). In this section, pharmacotherapy of each of these disorders is discussed in turn.

Separation Anxiety Disorder (School Phobia)

The psychotherapeutic and cognitive-behavioral tactics used by a therapist to treat children with separation anxiety disorder, including the symptoms of school phobia or school refusal, may sometimes be supplemented by a pharmacotherapy consultation and treatment. Often, an unresponsive case of separation anxiety disorder or school phobia is complicated by developmental or familial components that must be attended to as well. A fully defined and integrated multimodal treatment plan is often the most expeditious approach.

The two pharmacotherapeutic approaches most commonly employed to treat separation anxiety disorder associated with school refusal are the TCAs and the benzodiazepines (Sylvester and Kruesi 1994). The latter approach has been more typically used to treat overanxious states such as performance anxiety, although a recent study of clonazepam in childhood anxiety disorders emphasized the danger of disinhibition as a potential adverse effect (Graae et al. 1994). Benzodiazepines can also play a role in the treatment of school refusal or anticipatory anxiety (Bernstein and Borchardt 1991).

Recently, there has been a tendency to use SSRIs or TCAs (e.g., imipramine [Gittelman-Klein and Klein 1971]) for children with separation anxiety disorder, although an attempt to replicate the initial positive imipramine study failed to confirm that drug's overall benefits even though improvement was seen in some individuals (Klein et al. 1992). Because most controlled studies have failed to document a consistently positive response, Popper (1993) recommends that attention be given to comorbid conditions, concurrent stressors, and the secondary complications of truancy. He further advocates a multimodal treatment approach with a clearly defined, family-based cognitive-behavioral approach that uses goal setting, limit setting, and positive reinforcement.

It is in those children with a poor or limited response to multimodal psychotherapeutic treatment that a pharmacotherapy referral is especially indicated. If the techniques described in this chapter have been adopted, the pharmacotherapist will see a child and family already familiar with the concept of target symptoms and able to delineate the symptoms for which medication may be most useful. The family will have reviewed preexisting sensitivities to anxiety in the child's developmental history and will have considered the possible vulnerability within the family's history. As a result, the consultant's questions will be familiar and collaboration easier. Because the potential use of a medication trial may provoke further anxious responding on the part of parents or child, the preparation that has focused on managing the anxiety disorder with other techniques will have been quite useful. When pharmacotherapy is integrated with psychotherapy, parents and child are more likely to accept these approaches as complementary. This supports the family's coping skills.

Even when a specific youngster responds well to medication, parental limits are still needed. The parents may need guidance, too, in order to support their child's return to school, confrontation of associated developmental challenges, and fuller participation in peer-based activities. This caution is particularly germane in regard to consolidating the coping abilities and psychosocial competencies in childhood and adolescence. The family's fear that more serious dysfunction may disrupt the child's future can be diminished by the increased understanding and sense of efficacy that accompany psychoeducational and cognitive-behavioral interventions.

Panic Disorder

Clinicians must be alert to the early onset of panic disorder in children with a history of anxiety. From a pharmacotherapeutic standpoint, the TCAs and the benzodiazepines are considered effective treatments. There are as yet no well-controlled, double-blind studies to support their use in children, but such use is well established in adults (see Chapter 3), and a series of clinical reports have suggested that imipramine, desipramine, clonazepam, or alprazolam can be beneficial in children (Simeon and Ferguson 1987). Although considered a safe and promising approach in most children (Biederman 1987), clonazepam has been associated with occasional anger outbursts and disinhibition in some prepubertal children and adolescents (Reiter and Kutcher 1991).

During the symptom review with a child or adolescent patient and family, the distinctive symptoms of panic disorder are sought, with particular attention to whether panic attacks may also be tied to avoidance of school attendance or associated with other undesired activities.

Obsessive-Compulsive Disorder

The effectiveness of pharmacotherapy is more thoroughly demonstrated for obsessive-compulsive disorder than for any of the other childhood anxiety disorders. Treatment of children with the TCA clomipramine has been shown effective, and this result has been replicated (Flament et al. 1987; Leonard et al. 1991). The SSRIs fluoxetine (Leonard et al. 1993; Geller et al. 1995; Riddle et al. 1992), sertraline (March et al. 1994), and fluvoxamine (Apter et al. 1994) also appear effective in treating this disorder and may present a more easily tolerated spectrum of side effects. Variant forms of obsessive-compulsive disorder, such as trichotillomania, have likewise been suggested in case reports to be responsive to pharmacotherapy (Sheikha et al. 1993; Weller et al. 1989).

Although response to pharmacotherapy may be positive, the pervasiveness and seriousness of obsessive-compulsive disorder cannot be denied. Even in successful pharmacotherapy, symptoms tend to be reduced rather than eradicated. In view of this circumstance, Rapoport and colleagues (1993) argue for a psychoeducational and family-oriented approach, like the one advocated here, that minimizes secondary avoidance or social withdrawal, informs and strengthens family collaboration, and helps to normalize family life.

Preliminary empirical support for an integrated treatment approach has been offered by a recent study that combined sertraline pharmacotherapy with behavior therapy in children and adolescents with obsessive-compulsive disorder (March 1995; March et al. 1994).

Children or adolescents who present a clear symptom profile of obsessive-compulsive disorder should be informed of the availability of medication as a component of treatment. The risks and benefits of pharmacotherapy must be considered and discussed with the patient's parents or guardian(s). Pharmacotherapy may be of greatest value when placed within the context of a treatment program that includes concurrent behavioral and family interventions.

Attentional Disorders With Comorbid Anxiety and/or Depression

The frequent association of attentional disorders with comorbid anxious or depressive features has prompted study of these comorbid conditions in children. Although many patients with ADHD improve even on pharmacotherapy alone as a result of increased behavioral control and improved self-esteem, a number of children continue to have difficulties. Some of these respond quite well to TCAs (Ambrosini et al. 1993; Biederman et al. 1993a); however, the increased risk in overdose (Biggs et al. 1977) and the controversy regarding the cardiac safety of the TCAs have complicated the use of these agents. All TCAs are capable of affecting cardiac conduction (Puig-Antich et al. 1987), and they also share side effects that include postural hypotension, tachycardia, and systolic/diastolic hypertension. Their role in the causation of sudden death (Werry 1994), however, remains a matter of scientific controversy with little substantiation (Riddle et al. 1994).

Elective Mutism (Social Phobia/Avoidant Disorder)

For children with elective mutism (*selective mutism* in DSM-IV), a condition that some have speculated is a variant of social phobia (Black and Uhde 1992), treatment with a combination of psychotherapy, behavior therapy, and family therapy has been suggested to be efficacious (Labbe and Williamson 1984; Meyers 1984; Parker et al. 1960). An integrated multimodal program that combined all these elements has reported highly successful results (Krohn et al. 1992), although further validation is still required. One well-controlled study of fluoxetine is also available, although it is noteworthy that some subjects in this study responded significantly only after 3 months of pharmacotherapy (Black and Uhde 1994). This study and another recent report (Birmaher et al. 1994) bolster hopes that the SSRIs will acquire a valuable role in the treatment of childhood anxiety disorders.

▌ Conclusions

The principles of the cognitive-behavioral approach described in this chapter highlight four basic ingredients of a psychotherapeutic and psychoeducational approach to the treatment of anxiety disorders in children: 1) helping the child and parents achieve an understanding of the child's anxiety, 2) assisting in strengthening the child's coping skills, 3) showing the parents how to support the child's emotional needs and to set appropriate limits on the child's behavior, and 4) enhancing social and emotional understanding and problem solving within the family as a whole. Making books for and with children identifies specific coping strategies for the child or adolescent to use and engages the family in age-appropriate psychosocial problem solving and communication. This book-making technique creates a context in which psychopharmacological consultation can easily be integrated into a psychosocial treatment program.

∎ References

Achenbach T, Edelbrock C: Manual for the Child Behavior Checklist and Revised Child Behavior Profile. Burlington, VT, University of Vermont, Department of Psychiatry, 1983

Adamec RE, Stark-Adamec C: Kindling, in The Limbic System: Functional Organization and Clinical Disorders. Edited by Doane BK, Livingston KE. New York, Raven, 1986, pp 129–145

Aman M, Werry J: Methylphenidate and diazepam in severe reading retardation. Journal of the American Academy of Child Psychiatry 21:31–37, 1982

Ambrosini PJ, Bianchi MD, Rabinovich H, et al: Antidepressant treatments in children and adolescents, II: anxiety, physical and behavioral disorders. J Am Acad Child Adolesc Psychiatry 32:483–493, 1993

American Academy of Child and Adolescent Psychiatry: Guidelines for the clinical evaluation of child and adolescent sexual abuse (position statement). J Am Acad Child Adolesc Psychiatry 27:655–657, 1988

American Psychiatric Association: Diagnostic and Statistical Manual of Mental Disorders, 3rd Edition, Revised. Washington, DC, American Psychiatric Association, 1987

American Psychiatric Association: Diagnostic and Statistical Manual of Mental Disorders, 4th Edition. Washington, DC, American Psychiatric Association, 1994

Apter A, Ratzoni G, King RA, et al: Fluvoxamine open-label treatment of adolescent inpatients with obsessive-compulsive disorder or depression. J Am Acad Child Adolesc Psychiatry 33:342–348, 1994

Barlow DH: Cognitive-behavioral approaches to panic disorder and social phobia. Bull Menninger Clin (suppl):56:A14–A28, 1992

Bernstein GA, Borchardt CM: Anxiety disorders of childhood and adolescence: a critical review. J Am Acad Child Adolesc Psychiatry 30:519–532, 1991

Bernstein G, Garfinkel B: School phobia, the overlap of affective and anxiety disorders. Journal of the American Academy of Child Psychiatry 25:235–241, 1986

Bernstein G, Garfinkel B, Borchardt C: Comparative studies of pharmacotherapy for school refusal. J Am Acad Child Adolesc Psychiatry 29:773–781, 1990

Biederman J: Clonazepam in the treatment of prepubertal children with panic-like symptoms. J Clin Psychiatry 48:38–41, 1987

Biederman J: Psychopharmacology, in Textbook of Child and Adolescent Psychiatry. Edited by Weiner J. Washington, DC, American Psychiatric Press, 1991, pp 545–570

Biederman J, Rosenbaum JF, Hirshfeld DR, et al: Psychiatric correlates of behavioral inhibition in young children of parents with and without psychiatric disorders. Arch Gen Psychiatry 47:21–26, 1990

Biederman J, Newcorn J, Sprich S: Comorbidity of attention-deficit hyperactivity disorder with conduct, depressive, anxiety, and other disorders. Am J Psychiatry 148:564–577, 1991

Biederman J, Baldessarini RJ, Wright V, et al: A double-blind placebo-controlled study of desipramine in the treatment of ADD, III: lack of impact of comorbidity and family history factors on clinical response. J Am Acad Child Adolesc Psychiatry 32:199–204, 1993a

Biederman J, Rosenbaum J, Bolduc-Murphy E, et al: A 3-year follow-up of children with and without behavioral inhibition. J Am Acad Child Adolesc Psychiatry 32:814–821, 1993b

Biggs JT, Spiker DG, Petit JM, et al: Tricyclic antidepressant overdose. JAMA 238:135–138, 1977

Birmaher B, Waterman GS, Ryan N, et al: Fluoxetine for childhood anxiety disorders. J Am Acad Child Adolesc Psychiatry 33:993–999, 1994

Black B, Uhde T: Elective mutism as a variant of social phobia. J Am Acad Child Adolesc Psychiatry 31:1091–1094, 1992

Black B, Uhde T: Treatment of elective mutism with fluoxetine: a double-blind, placebo-controlled study. J Am Acad Child Adolesc Psychiatry 33:1000–1006, 1994

Breier A, Charney DS, Heninger GR: Major depression in patients with agoraphobia and panic disorder. Arch Gen Psychiatry 41:1129–1135, 1984

Brown R, Kaslow N, Hazzard A, et al: Psychiatric and family functioning in children with leukemia and their parents. J Am Acad Child Adolesc Psychiatry 31:495–502, 1992

Burns DD: The Feeling Good Handbook. New York, Plume Books, 1990

Carlson C, Figueroa R, Lahey B: Behavior therapy for childhood anxiety disorders, in Anxiety Disorders of Childhood. Edited by Gittelman R. New York, Guilford, 1986, pp 204–232

Coffey BJ: Anxiolytics for children and adolescents: traditional and new drugs. Journal of Child and Adolescent Psychopharmacology 1:57–83, 1990

Cohen DJ, Paul R, Volkmar FR: Issues in the classification of pervasive developmental disorders and associated conditions, in Handbook of Autism and Pervasive Developmental Disorders. Edited by Cohen DJ, Donellan A. New York, Wiley, 1987, pp 20–40

Conners CK: A teacher rating scale for use in drug studies with children. Am J Psychiatry 126:884–888, 1969

Conners CK: Rating scales for use in drug studies with children. Psychopharmacol Bull 9:24–84, 1973

Cotton N: The deadly combination: adolescence and mental illness. Paper presented at the Harvard Medical School Continuing Education Conference, Cambridge, MA, February 1994

DeVeaugh-Geiss J, Moroz G, Biederman J, et al: Clomipramine hydrochloride in childhood and adolescent obsessive-compulsive disorder: a multicenter trial. J Am Acad Child Adolesc Psychiatry 31:45–49, 1992

Di Leo J: Children's Drawings as Diagnostic Aids. New York, Brunner/Mazel, 1973

DuPaul GJ, Barkley RA, McMurray MB: Response of children with ADHD to methylphenidate: interaction with internalizing symptoms. J Am Acad Child Adolesc Psychiatry 33:894–903, 1994

Flament M, Rapoport JL, Berg C, et al: Clomipramine treatment of childhood obsessive-compulsive disorder. Arch Gen Psychiatry 42:977–983, 1987

Francis G, Last C, Strauss C: Avoidant disorder and social phobia in children and adolescents. J Am Acad Child Adolesc Psychiatry 31:1087–1089, 1992

Free N, Winget C, Whitman R: Separation anxiety in panic disorder. Am J Psychiatry 150:595–599, 1993

Freud S: Analysis of a phobia in a five-year-old boy (1909), in Standard Edition of the Complete Psychological Works of Sigmund Freud, Vol 10. Translated and edited by Strachey J. London, Hogarth Press, 1955, pp 1–149

Gabbard G: Psychodynamics of panic disorder and social phobia. Bull Menninger Clin 56 (suppl A):A3–A13, 1992

Geller DA, Biederman J, Reed Ed, et al: Similarities in response to fluoxetine in the treatment of children and adolescents with obsessive-compulsive disorder. J Am Acad Child Adolesc Psychiatry 34:36–44, 1995

Gilham R: Refractory epilepsy: an evaluation of psychological methods in outpatient management. Epilepsia 31:427–432, 1990

Gittelman-Klein R, Klein DF: Controlled imipramine treatment of school phobia. Arch Gen Psychiatry 25:204–207, 1971

Goldfried M: Systematic desensitization as training in self-control. J Consult Clin Psychol 37:228–234, 1971

Gorman JM, Liebowitz MR, Fyer AJ, et al: A neuroanatomical hypothesis for panic disorder. Am J Psychiatry 146:148–161, 1989

Graae F, Milner J, Rizzotto L, et al: Clonazepam in childhood anxiety disorders. J Am Acad Child Adolesc Psychiatry 33:372–376, 1994

Helfer RE: Child abuse and neglect: the diagnostic process and treatment programs (DHEW Publ No OHD-75-69). Washington, DC, U.S. Department of Health, Education, and Welfare, 1975

Jan JE, Ziegler RG, Erba G: Does Your Child Have Epilepsy? Austin, TX, Pro-Ed, 1991

Jensen P, Shervette R, Xenakis S, et al: Anxiety and depressive disorders in attention-deficit disorder with hyperactivity: new findings. Am J Psychiatry 150:1203–1209, 1993

Jones MC: The elimination of children's fears. Journal of Experimental Psychology 7:382–390, 1924

Joorabchi B: Expressions of the hyperventilation syndrome in childhood: studies in the management, including an evaluation of the effectiveness of propranolol. Clin Pediatr (Phila) 16:1110–1115, 1977

Kagan J, Reznick JS, Snidman N: Biological basis of childhood shyness. Science 240:167–171, 1988

Kashani JH, Orvaschel H: A community study of anxiety in children and adolescents. Am J Psychiatry 147:313–318, 1990

Kashani JH, Anasseril ED, Dandoy AC, et al: Family violence: impact on children. J Am Acad Child Adolesc Psychiatry 31:181–189, 1992

Keller MB, Lavori PW, Wunder J, et al: Chronic course of anxiety disorders in children and adolescents. J Am Acad Child Adolesc Psychiatry 31:595–599, 1992

Kiser LJ, Heston J, Millsap PA, et al: Physical and sexual abuse in childhood: relationship with post-traumatic stress disorder. J Am Acad Child Adolesc Psychiatry 30:776–783, 1991

Klein R, Koplewicz H, Kanner A: Imipramine treatment of children with separation anxiety disorder. J Am Acad Child Adolesc Psychiatry 31:21–28, 1992

Koeppen AS: Relaxation training for children. Elementary School Guidance and Counseling 9:521–528, 1974

Krohn D, Weckstein S, Wright H: A study of the effectiveness of a specific treatment for elective mutism. J Am Acad Child Adolesc Psychiatry 31:711–718, 1992

Kutcher SP, MacKenzie S: Successful clonazepam treatment of adolescents with panic disorder. J Clin Psychopharmacol 8:922–924, 1988

Labbe EE, Williamson DA: Behavioral treatment of elective mutism: a review of the literature. Clinical Psychology Review 4:273–294, 1984

Last C, Perrin S, Hersen M, et al: DSM-III-R anxiety disorders in children: sociodemographic and clinical characteristics. J Am Acad Child Adolesc Psychiatry 31:1070–1076, 1992

Lenane MC, Swedo SE, Rapoport JL, et al: Rates of obsessive-compulsive disorder in first-degree relatives of patients with trichotillomania: a research note. Journal of Clinical Psychology and Psychiatry and Allied Disciplines 33:925–933, 1992

Leonard HL, Swedo SE, Rapoport JL, et al: Treatment of obsessive-compulsive disorder with clomipramine and desipramine in children and adolescents: a double-blind crossover comparison. Arch Gen Psychiatry 46:1088–1092, 1989

Leonard HL, Swedo SE, Lenane MC, et al: A double-blind desipramine substitution during long-term clomipramine treatment in children and adolescents with obsessive-compulsive disorder. Arch Gen Psychiatry 48:922–926, 1991

Leonard HL, Swedo SE, Lenane MC, et al: A 2- to 7-year follow-up study of 54 obsessive-compulsive children and adolescents. Arch Gen Psychiatry 50:429–439, 1993

Lewis D: From abuse to violence: psychophysiological consequences of maltreatment. J Am Acad Child Adolesc Psychiatry 31:383–391, 1992

Livingston R: Anxiety disorders, in A Comprehensive Textbook of Child Psychiatry. Edited by Lewis M. Baltimore, MD, Williams & Wilkins, 1991, pp 673–684

Lothman D, Pianta R: Role of child-mother interaction in predicting competence of children with epilepsy. Epilepsia 34:658–669, 1993

Lyman DR, Selman RL: Peer conflict in pair therapy: clinical and developmental analyses. New Dir Child Dev 29:85–102, 1985

Manassis K, Bradley S, Goldberg S, et al: Attachment in mothers with anxiety disorders and their children. J Am Acad Child Adolesc Psychiatry 33:1106–1113, 1994

March JS: Cognitive-behavioral psychotherapy for children and adolescents with OCD: a review and recommendations for treatment. J Am Acad Child Adolesc Psychiatry 34:7–18, 1995

March JS, Mulle K, Herbel B: Behavioral psychotherapy for children and adolescents with obsessive-compulsive disorder: an open trial of a new protocol-driven treatment package. J Am Acad Child Adolesc Psychiatry 33:333–341, 1994

Messer SC, Beidel DC: Psychosocial correlates of childhood anxiety disorders. J Am Acad Child Adolesc Psychiatry 33:975–983, 1994

Meyers SV: Elective mutism in children: a family systems approach. Am J Family Therapy 12:39–45, 1984

Moreau D, Weissman M: Panic disorder in children and adolescents: a review. Am J Psychiatry 149:1306–1314, 1992

National Institute of Mental Health: Understanding panic disorder (NIH Publ No 93-3509). Rockville, MD, U.S. Department of Health and Human Services, 1993

Parker EB, Eisen TF, Throckmorton MC: Social casework with elementary school children who do not talk in school. Soc Work 5:64–70, 1960

Plizka SR: Comorbidity of attention-deficit hyperactivity disorder and overanxious disorder. J Am Acad Child Adolesc Psychiatry 31:197–203, 1992

Popper CW: Psychopharmacologic treatment of anxiety disorders in adolescents and children. J Clin Psychiatry 54 (5, suppl):52–63, 1993

Puig-Antich J, Perel JM, Lupatkin W, et al: Imipramine in prepubertal major depressive disorders. Arch Gen Psychiatry 44:81–89, 1987

Ramirez S, Kratochwill T, Morris R: Childhood anxiety disorders, in Anxiety and Stress Disorders: Cognitive-Behavioral Assessment and Treatment. Edited by Michelson L, Ascher LM. New York, Guilford, 1987, pp 149–175

Rapoport J, Leonard H, Swedo S, et al: Obsessive-compulsive disorder in children and adolescents: issues in management. J Clin Psychiatry 54 (6, suppl):24–29, 1993

Reiter S, Kutcher SP: Disinhibition and anger outbursts in adolescents treated with clonazepam (letter). J Clin Psychopharmacol 11:268, 1991

Riddle MA, Scahill L, King RA, et al: Double-blind, crossover trial of fluoxetine and placebo in children and adolescents with obsessive-compulsive disorder. J Am Acad Child Adolesc Psychiatry 31:1062–1069, 1992

Riddle MA, Geller B, Ryan N: The safety of desipramine (letter to editor). J Am Acad Child Adolesc Psychiatry 33:589–590, 1994

Rosenbaum JF, Biederman J, Bolduc EA, et al: Comorbidity of parental anxiety disorders as risk for childhood-onset anxiety in inhibited children. Am J Psychiatry 149:475–481, 1992

Scheafer CE: Therapeutic Use of Child's Play. New York, Jason Aronson, 1976

Shear MK, Cooper AM, Klerman GL, et al: A psychodynamic model of panic disorder. Am J Psychiatry 150:859–866, 1993

Sheehan DV, Sheehan KE, Minichiello WE: Age of onset of phobic disorders: a reevaluation. Compr Psychiatry 22:535–544, 1981

Sheikha SH, Wagner KD, Wagner RF Jr: Fluoxetine treatment of trichotillomania and depression in a prepubertal child. Cutis 51:50–52, 1993

Simeon J, Ferguson H: Alprazolam effects in children with anxiety disorders. Can J Psychiatry 40:1228–1231, 1987

Spitzer R, Skodol A, Gibbon M, et al: DSM-III Casebook. Washington, DC, American Psychiatric Press, 1981

Steingard R: Psychopharmacology perspectives: response to case presentations in Child Psychotherapy Conference. Sponsored by Harvard Medical School Department of Continuing Education. Boston, MA, June 1993

Swedo SE, Leonard HL: Childhood movement disorders and obsessive-compulsive disorder. J Clin Psychiatry 55 (3, suppl):32–37, 1994

Sylvester C, Kruesi M: Child and adolescent psychopharmacotherapy: progress and pitfalls. Psychiatric Annals 24:83–90, 1994

Thomas A, Chess S: Temperament and Development. New York, Brunner/Mazel, 1977

Thyer BA, Parris RT, Curtis GC, et al: Ages of onset of DSM-III anxiety disorders. Compr Psychiatry 26:113–122, 1985

Turecki S, with Tonner L: The Difficult Child. New York, Bantam Books, 1985

Verhulst FC, van der Ende J: Six-year developmental course of internalizing and externalizing problem behaviors. J Am Acad Child Adolesc Psychiatry 31:924–931, 1992

Watson JB, Rayner R: Conditioned emotional reaction. Journal of Experimental Psychology 3:1–14, 1920

Wechsler D: Manual for Wechsler Intelligence Scale for Children, 3rd Edition (WISC-III). San Antonio, TX, Psychological Corporation, 1991

Weller EB, Weller RA, Carr S: Imipramine treatment of trichotillomania and coexisting depression in a 7-year-old. J Am Acad Child Adolesc Psychiatry 28:952–953, 1989

Werry JS: The safety of desipramine (letter). J Am Acad Child Adolesc Psychiatry 33:588–589, 1994

Ziegler R: Task-focused therapy with children and families. Am J Psychother 34:107–118, 1980

Ziegler R: Impairments of control and competence in epileptic children and their families. Epilepsia 22:339–346, 1981

Ziegler R: Homemade Books to Help Kids Cope: A Guide for Parents and Professionals. New York, Magination Press (Brunner/Mazel), 1992

Ziegler R, Holden L: Focused child and family therapy for children with learning disabilities and attentional disorders. Am J Orthopsychiatry 58:192–210, 1988

Medical Causes of Anxiety: A Guide to Recognition

Douglas H. Hughes, M.D.

O ne of the greatest diagnostic challenges in treating patients who complain of anxiety is to differentiate conditions that require medical attention from those that are primarily psychosocial in nature. Because some medical disorders that present with symptoms of anxiety are life-threatening, this differentiation cannot always await a leisurely diagnostic process. The conscientious psychotherapist, recognizing that anxiety is a nonspecific symptom, considers possible medical conditions both in new patients and in current patients who develop new symptoms. My purpose in this chapter is to familiarize mental health clinicians with the autonomic nervous system's role in the physiology of anxiety, the frequent comorbidity of anxiety disorders with substance abuse or other factors predisposing to poor physical health, guidelines for assessing the presence of organic causes of anxiety, and a spectrum of physical disorders capable of producing anxiety symptoms. The organic syndromes examined in greater detail are substance abuse, anxiety related to the use of prescribed medications, acquired immunodeficiency syndrome (AIDS), hyperthyroidism, hypoglycemia, and pheochromocytoma.

■ Review of the Autonomic Nervous System's Role in Anxiety Symptoms

The autonomic nervous system, a component of the central nervous system (CNS) that is responsible for maintaining bodily function despite changing internal and external conditions, can be divided into two major subsystems: the sympathetic and the parasympathetic systems. Each of these plays a major role in the experience of anxiety. A review of the autonomic nervous system's functioning illustrates how either medical or psychosocial factors can ultimately lead to identical anxiety symptoms.

Sympathetic System

The massive activation of the sympathetic system that occurs in response to severe danger has been called the "fight or flight" response (Lefkowitz et al. 1990, p. 88). This response serves to provide the body with an immediate burst of energy by speeding up the heart, increasing blood pressure, increasing oxygenation of skeletal muscle, expanding the lungs, dilating the pupils, and increasing the level of glucose in the blood. The subjective internal state accompanying these changes is one of arousal, anxiety, or fear. The sympathetic system can be activated to a lesser degree, too, leading to partial or intermittent activity with intensity related to environmental circumstances. Functioning normally, this response pattern allows for fine-tuning of an individual's response to his or her surroundings. When the sympathetic system is triggered excessively or inappropriately, however, the individual undergoes a strong and distressing fight-or-flight response that is experienced as anxiety with associated physical changes (see Table 8–1) (Lefkowitz et al. 1990).

Parasympathetic System

The primary functions of the parasympathetic system are to promote resting-organ function and to conserve energy. Parasympathetic cardiac effects include decreased heart rate and lowered blood pressure. The gastrointestinal effects include stimulation of gastric and intestinal secretions, peristalsis, enhanced absorption of nutrients, and voiding of the rectum. The parasympathetic system usually discharges in a controlled and modulated manner. When it discharges excessively, the result is a chaotic and disorganized disruption of normal functioning (see Table 8–1) (Lefkowitz et al. 1990). The parasympathetic state is typically regarded as antithetical to anxiety, although there are important exceptions: motion sickness, vasovagal syncope, and postural hypotension are examples of conditions in which parasympathetic hyperfunction can lead to anxiety

Table 8–1.   End-organ response to sympathetic and parasympathetic activation

End organ	Sympathetic activation	Parasympathetic activation
Pupil	Dilate	Contract
Heart	Increase rate	Decrease rate
Lung muscles	Relax (expand)	Contract
Lung secretion	Decrease	Increase
Gastrointestinal motility	Decrease	Increase
Blood vessels:		
Skin	Contract	Dilate
Cerebral	Contract	Dilate
Mucosa	Contract	Dilate

Source.   Adapted from Lefkowitz et al. 1990, pp. 89–90.

accompanied by nausea, vomiting, and marked drops in resting blood pressure (Berkow 1992).

The DSM-IV (American Psychiatric Association 1994) anxiety disorders prominently feature signs and symptoms of autonomic hyperfunction. In both generalized anxiety disorder and panic disorder, hyperarousal is frequently and spontaneously present. In the phobic disorders or in posttraumatic stress disorder, signs and symptoms of hyperarousal are experienced when the patient confronts a feared situation. In obsessive-compulsive disorder, these signs and symptoms are manifested when the patient resists obsessing or performing compulsive activities (American Psychiatric Association 1994).

▌ Comorbidity and Anxiety

Even when a primary physical cause for anxiety is not suspected, anxiety is often accompanied by complicating factors with implications for an individual's physical health. Individuals who suffer from panic disorder, for example, show a substantially higher risk both of poor physical health and of ethanol or other drug abuse (Massion et al. 1993). The presence of panic disorder is also associated with an increased risk for suicide attempts and completed suicides (Weissman et al. 1984).

Related findings have been reported with respect to generalized anxiety disorder from two large-scale, population-based studies: the Harvard/Brown Anxiety Research Program (Massion et al. 1993) and the Epidemiologic Catchment Area (ECA) survey (Myers et al. 1984). Subjects with generalized anxiety disorder had a prevalence of lifetime ethanol abuse of about 26% (25% and 27%, respectively, in the Harvard/Brown and the ECA studies), and a history of other substance abuse of about 17% (15% and 18%). Self-ratings of physical health as "fair" or "poor" ranged from 23% to 35% (Massion et al. 1993). In another study (Breslau et al. 1993), the presence of anxiety was correlated with smoking and nicotine dependence.

▌ Initial Evaluation of the Anxious Patient

Some general guidelines can be recommended to assist clinicians in determining which anxious patients to refer for further medical evaluation. First, it is recommended that a recent medical evaluation be documented or a new one performed for any patient experiencing severe psychological distress (Saklad 1985). Even when organic illness appears less likely, it is prudent to request a physical examination for any patient who has not had one within the past year or within 6 months prior to the onset of anxiety. Early consideration of consultation is of particular importance because psychotherapists' levels of expertise, familiarity, and comfort with medical issues vary greatly. A collegial relationship with a physician or nurse practitioner can facilitate referral of appropriate cases and provide a resource for discussion of ambiguous cases.

The basic medical assessment, usually performed by a consulting physician or advanced-practice nurse, includes a comprehensive history. In addition to current and past psychiatric symptomatology, the evaluator notes current and past medical illnesses, prescribed medications, and recreational drug use. The family's psychiatric and medical history can provide additional insight. Initial physical examination focuses on obvious signs of autonomic hyperarousal such as abnormal vital signs (temperature, blood pressure, pulse, and respiratory rate) and may include screening laboratory tests such as a complete blood count, blood and urine toxicology screens, thyroid function screen, electrolytes, renal function tests, blood glucose measurement, and an electrocardiogram (ECG). If this basic assessment reveals no evidence suggesting medical illness, then no further tests may be required. If the diagnosis remains in question or the patient fails to improve as expected, further evaluation should be considered. Patients in ongoing treatment may need medical reassessment for newly arising symptoms. It may be difficult to determine, for example, whether chronic mental illness, substance abuse, or a medical disorder has caused or exacerbated anxiety at a specific moment in an individual with paranoid schizophrenia, long-standing alcohol abuse, and ischemic heart disease. When doubt remains, further examination or periodic reassessment may provide valuable insight.

A more extensive physical evaluation of the anxious patient could include neurological assessment (by psychiatrist, internist or primary care physician, nurse, or consulting neurologist) and/or further laboratory tests. The clinical examination would include testing of orientation to person, place, time, and situation; memory for recent and remote events; speech, which may be dysarthric when neurological impairment or drug intoxication are present; gait, which is often impaired with neurological disease or intoxication; and visual fields and pupillary responses. More extensive laboratory evaluation might include chest X ray, magnetic resonance imaging (MRI) or computed tomography (CT) scan, spinal lumbar puncture with examination of cerebrospinal fluid, 24-hour urine catecholamine measurement, human immunodeficiency virus (HIV) testing, T-lymphocyte count, or electroencephalogram (EEG).

Some general caveats can be offered. When an anxious patient presents with no premorbid psychiatric history, consideration of organicity is important. An organic etiology for anxiety is more likely in patients whose anxiety began after age 40 and cannot be explained psychosocially, although the presence of psychosocial stressors does not eliminate the possibility of a concurrent medical disorder. Furthermore, a recent medical examination also does not rule out the possibility of a medical disorder, because many patients are referred for mental health treatment by physicians who have overlooked primarily physical causes of mental symptoms (Koranyi 1979).

▌ Specific Substances and Medical Disorders That Cause Anxiety

The complete list of substances and medical disorders that can cause or contribute to anxiety is too lengthy to enumerate here. For mental health clinicians, the diagnostic challenge with anxious patients is to divert those who are medically ill toward appropriate treatments, particularly when a life-threatening condition is present. In the following section I use case examples to illustrate a few of these conditions. The disorders to be discussed are more-or-less common ones with potentially serious outcomes: substance abuse, adverse effects of prescribed medications, AIDS, hyperthyroidism, hypoglycemia, and pheochromocytoma.

Anxiety Resulting From Use of Recreational or Prescribed Drugs

This section contains three parts: first, anxiety-producing recreational drugs are discussed. Next, a group of anxiety-inducing therapeutic medications is reviewed. Finally, guidelines are offered for the use of toxicology screens.

Anxiety-Producing Recreational Drugs

Recent statistics from the U.S. Alcohol, Drug Abuse and Mental Health Administration (Ellis 1993) may provide some perspective on the prevalence of drug abuse. According to this source, every day in the United States, 20 people will die as a result of using illicit drugs. During that same day, 350 Americans will expire as a direct or indirect consequence of ethanol ingestion—either in car accidents or from cirrhosis or other ethanol-related illnesses. Furthermore, more than 1,000 people die daily from diseases related to nicotine addiction (Kong 1990). The primary psychiatric anxiety disorders co-occur frequently with substance abuse or dependence. Paradoxically, many people are believed to "self-medicate" (Khantzian 1985) the symptoms of a primary anxiety disorder with drugs that, during withdrawal, are themselves capable of producing anxiety symptoms.

Legal intoxicants. *Nicotine,* the active ingredient in tobacco preparations, is a powerful and ubiquitous intoxicant. Its short-term effects may appear beneficial, given that it facilitates concentration and memory, mitigates aggressive behavior, and assists with weight loss. Nicotine apparently works as an appetite suppressant, especially for sweeter-tasting food, which accounts for the finding that the average smoker weighs 5–10 pounds less than the average nonsmoker (Jaffe 1990). Nicotine may also increase energy expenditure both at rest and during exercise. As Glassman (1993) speculated, "it seems logical that patients with high levels of anxiety or with anxiety disorders would smoke more because smokers regularly report that nicotine diminishes anxiety" (p. 548).

Smokers rapidly develop tolerance to and dependence on nicotine (Jaffe 1990). The signs and symptoms of nicotine withdrawal resemble those of several other anxiety disorders, and include restlessness, anxiety, irritability, and changes in appetite (American Psychiatric Association 1994).

Caffeine, another legal and widely available intoxicant, is found in many popular beverages (see Table 8–2). A cup of brewed coffee contains roughly 112 mg of caffeine, approximately 50% more caffeine than the average amount contained in a cup of instant coffee. A serving of cola or tea contains less than half the amount of caffeine found in a cup of brewed coffee. In the United States, the average adult consumes between 170 and 200 mg of caffeine per day (Iserson 1990; Syed 1976).

At doses exceeding 250 mg/day, symptoms of caffeine intoxication can occur, including restlessness, nervousness, excitement, insomnia, tachycardia, and psychomotor agitation (American Psy-

Table 8–2.   Caffeine content of some common beverages

Beverage	Caffeine content
Coffee, brewed	85–139 mg/cup
Coffee, instant	60–99 mg/cup
Tea, caffeinated	30–75 mg/cup
Cola, caffeinated	40–60 mg/12 oz

Source.   Adapted from Syed 1976, p. 568, and Iserson 1990, p. 869.

chiatric Association 1994). Most caffeine is consumed in the form of coffee (Clemeatz and Dailey 1988), and the coffee bean contains acidic oils that can irritate the stomach and intestines, leading also to diarrhea. At levels of daily consumption exceeding 400 mg and continuing for at least 1 week, some degree of tolerance and dependence can be expected to occur (Rall 1990). Because the use of caffeine is such a socially accepted custom, many consumers and clinicians fail either to classify it as an intoxicant or to take it into account in their psychological or pharmacological treatment plans.

Withdrawal from caffeine, too, can be associated with anxiety, often accompanied by fatigue and headaches. These symptoms begin within 12–24 hours after stopping (or significantly reducing) caffeine intake. They may persist for 2–7 days (Rall 1990).

Patients who already suffer from panic disorder may be particularly sensitive to the effects of caffeine. In one study, the majority of panic disorder subjects receiving doses of caffeine that resulted in plasma concentrations of about 8 µg/ml experienced anxiety, fear, and other symptoms characteristic of their panic attacks (Charney et al. 1985).

Ethanol ("alcohol") is abused by an estimated 7% of the adult population of the United States. Absorbed rapidly from the gastro-intestinal tract and from there into the CNS, ethanol produces a variety of behavioral and neurological changes within minutes of its ingestion. Mood can become anxious or depressed, with accompanying autonomic disturbances (Diamond 1992). Five ounces of wine, 12 ounces of beer, or 1.5 ounces of hard liquor (80-proof) will raise the serum ethanol level approximately 12 mg/deciliter (dl) within 30–45 minutes. At a level of 100 mg/dl, judgment and coordination are often impaired and most states recognize the presence of legal intoxication. An average liver will remove ethanol from the bloodstream and lower the blood ethanol level at a rate of 15–25 mg/dl per hour (Holbrook and Aghababian 1992).

Withdrawal from ethanol can be even more dangerous than intoxication, leading at times to fatal outcomes. Ethanol withdrawal may produce minor anxiety symptoms or a range of increasingly severe neurological disturbances (see Chapter 9). The most common withdrawal symptom is tremulousness, beginning about 6 hours after the last drink (Diamond 1992). Often associated with irritability, this state can appear indistinguishable from an anxiety disorder.

Illicit drugs.   An estimated 1–2 million Americans are dependent on *cocaine,* and 22 million have experimented with the drug (Higgins et al. 1991). Crack, the smoked freebase form of cocaine, is the most popular form of cocaine among abusers. It enters the bloodstream through the lungs and passes into the brain in less than 10 seconds. The euphoric effects are intensified and compressed into a few minutes, followed by dysphoria, anxiety, and craving for more of the drug. The anxiety can be particularly severe with inhaled (smoked) and intravenous routes of administration ("Crack," *Medical Letter* 1986). Anxiety and/or irritability can occur during or after cocaine intoxication, thus encouraging secondary abuse of ethanol or anxiolytics (Gawin and Ellinwood 1988). The results of chronic cocaine use can be difficult to differentiate from a functional paranoid disorder or an anxiety disorder without obtaining an accurate and comprehensive history. Furthermore, studies have associated cocaine abuse with kindling of autonomous panic disorder (McLellan et al. 1979) that can persist even in the absence of further cocaine use (Gawin and Ellinwood 1988). Although the number of cocaine users seeking treatment rose markedly in the 1980s, relapse rates remain high, and 30%–80% of patients drop out of treatment programs (Higgins et al. 1991). Pharmacotherapy may have a role in treating both drug craving and anxiety symptoms in cocaine abusers (Higgins et al. 1991).

Phencyclidine (PCP) can produce an extreme subjective anxiety associated with physical signs, including rotatory oscillation of the eyes, ataxia, bizarre facial grimacing, and a pronounced startle response. The intensity of intoxication is dose related, and drug-induced effects last 3–4 hours. The drug is detectable in the blood for several hours only, but can be detected in the urine for a longer period. PCP delirium can begin even as long as 1 week after discontinuation of use, and may last a week or more (Jaffe 1990). PCP use peaked in the mid-1970s, when the drug was used occasionally by an estimated 7 million Americans and taken at least once per week by as many as 1 million Americans (Aniline and Pitts 1982).

Stimulants, including amphetamines, methylphenidate, and others, remain popular drugs of abuse as well as therapeutic agents prescribed for the treatment of narcolepsy or attention-deficit/hyperactivity disorder (ADHD) or as a treatment alternative or adjunct in some cases of depression. Stimulants can cause a range of anxiety symptoms resulting from sympathetic hyperarousal, including tremor, anxiety, nausea, and vomiting. These drugs have also been reported to induce psychotic reactions (Hoffman and Lefkowitz 1990). Powerful new synthetic agents such as Ice and Ecstasy (methylenedioxymethamphetamine [MDMA], also "XTC") are becoming increasingly available. Ecstasy can cause destructive physical effects, including hyperthermia, muscle destruction, acute renal failure, hepatotoxicity, cardiac arrhythmias, and convulsions (Henry et al. 1992).

Anabolic steroid abuse has been associated with mood instability, irritability, and hostility that can resemble an anxiety disorder or psychogenic rage attacks (Su et al. 1993). The correct diagnosis may be difficult to discern when the presence of steroid abuse is disguised as "rage attacks." These drugs are most commonly abused by males of high school or college age, who take them to increase muscle mass for sports or appearance. Steroid abuse is not rare: of 1,881 Georgia high school students who answered a survey, 6.5% of the boys and 1.9% of the girls reported using steroids. Of incidental interest, 25% of those who used steroids reported having shared needles within the previous 30 days. There were also significant associations of steroid abuse with use of marijuana or cocaine (Durant et al. 1993). Medical complications of anabolic steroid abuse include hypertension, liver damage, and acne (Ishak 1979).

Anxiety-Producing Prescribed Medications

Among the many *prescribed medications* that have been associated with the production or aggravation of anxiety symptoms are the benzodiazepines, certain narcotic analgesics (e.g., meperidine), neuroleptics, corticosteroids, bronchodilators, and antidepressants. *Benzodiazepines* can produce in some people an idiosyncratic disinhibition that can be mistaken for primary rage or anxiety (Rosenbaum et al. 1984). It is important to recognize this adverse reaction so as to avoid worsening the situation in an attempt to relieve the symptoms by increasing the medication dosage. *Meperidine,* a powerful narcotic analgesic, can cause a paradoxical reaction of agitation, characterized by tremors, muscle twitches, and hyperactive reflexes (Jaffe and Martin 1990). *Neuroleptics* can produce akathisia, a syndrome of motor restlessness easily mistaken for primary anxiety. The distinction is an important one, because a mistaken diagnosis can lead to a counterproductive increase in neuroleptic dosage. Akathisia is particularly common with the higher-potency neuroleptics such as haloperidol, fluphenazine, trifluoperazine, or thiothixene. When a patient whose neuroleptic medication has recently been increased experiences an exacerbation of his or her anxiety symptoms, akathisia should be one of the potential causes considered (Miller and Jankovic 1990).

Corticosteroid treatment, frequently prescribed to suppress an inflammatory response or to counteract adrenal insufficiency, often is accompanied by anxiety symptoms and other behavioral disturbances. The anxiety can be observed with acute treatment, during the maintenance phase, or following withdrawal of the medication. Prolonged use of corticosteroids also produces physical changes such as hirsutism, central obesity, thin extremities, and a rounded face (Haynes 1990).

Bronchodilators, used in the treatment of asthma or chronic obstructive lung disease, have been associated with symptoms and signs of anxiety, including subjective mood changes, tachycardia, and tremulousness. They are often administered in aerosol form and produce rapid physiological effects. On occasion, patients who have not been advised of these potential adverse effects present with a confusing clinical picture that may easily be mistaken for another anxiety disorder (Rall 1990).

Antidepressant medications, usually anxiolytic in their effects, can sometimes produce undesired symptoms of anxiety. The more stimulating tricyclic antidepressants (TCAs), such as desipramine, and the dopamine reuptake blocker bupropion can cause subjective anxiety accompanied by autonomic symptoms. The TCAs can induce tachycardia, lightheadedness, palpitations, and dry mouth (Pollack and Rosenbaum 1987), and fluoxetine (and possibly the other serotonin reuptake–inhibiting antidepressants) can cause an akathisia-like, dose-related anxiety (Altamura et al. 1988). Because the antidepressants vary in their anxiogenic effects from person to person, an anxious reaction to an antidepressant may respond to a decrease in dosage, the addition of an anxiolytic drug, or a change to a different antidepressant. Abrupt withdrawal from TCAs has also been noted to produce anxiety symptoms (Dilsaver et al. 1983). More recently, withdrawal symptoms including anxiety have been attributed to discontinuation of serotonin reuptake inhibitors.

The Use of Toxicology Screens

Toxicology screens ("drug screens") can be used to help verify a diagnosis of substance abuse or intoxication. A variety of assay methods are in use; some of these merely indicate the presence of a substance, whereas others quantify the substance's concentration in the blood. Toxicology screens may be comprehensive, including more than 40 drugs, or limited to one or two substances. Preliminary results are often reported within an hour, with confirmation available within several hours.

Toxicology screens can be performed on serum, urine, or gastric samples. Serum samples, the most frequently ordered, allow determination of quantitative results. A urine screen, however, detects many additional substances of abuse—such as cocaine, amphetamines, narcotics, and cannabis—more sensitively. With a special technique, acidification of the urine, minuscule quantities of PCP can be detected. Yield and accuracy improve when both urine and serum samples are submitted for analysis. Gastric samples may be of particular value when a recent overdose is suspected, and gastric aspirates may contain larger amounts of the intoxicating substance (Haddad and Roberts 1990).

The usefulness of drug screens, unfortunately, is diminished by their limitations. Many substances, including lithium, heavy metals, and volatile hydrocarbons, are not routinely measured and require specific tests. Even when general categories are tested, specific members of that category may not be included in the assay. Most toxicology screens, for example, test for "benzodiazepines," yet few newer agents such as alprazolam (Xanax) are detected in these screens (Haddad and Roberts 1990). A patient intoxicated with alprazolam, therefore, might show a misleadingly negative drug screen result. There is also a high margin of error for drug screens, so that experts recommend confirmation by retesting and interpretation of results in light of an individual's clinical history and interview (Hoyt et al. 1987).

The following case example illustrates some of the difficulties in recognizing substance abuse as a covert cause of anxiety:

> Mr. A, a thin 24-year-old with chronic paranoid schizophrenia who had received weekly supportive outpatient psychotherapy for 2 years, complained of new anxiety symptoms. He stated that several times a week he had discrete periods of anxiety characterized by a racing heart, sweating palms, shortness of breath, and slight nausea. For the past 2 years, he had been treated with haloperidol 10 mg once per day and benztropine 2 mg twice per day. Mr. A drank more than 4 liters of diet cola per day and two beers per night, but denied that ethanol was a problem in his life. Although he denied having used any additional recreational drugs during the preceding 2 years, he admitted to having previously tried many types of recreational drugs. He was preoccupied with his weight.
>
> Initially, Mr. A refused random urine drug screens. Later, when he agreed, these tests revealed the presence of amphetamines. When confronted with this result, Mr. A admitted to using amphetamines but adamantly insisted that they were to lose weight and not to get high. With cessation of amphetamine use, Mr. A's anxiety diminished despite his continued use of large quantities of caffeinated diet cola.

Anxiety-Inducing Medical Disorders

From the extensive list of medical disorders capable of causing anxiety symptoms, a few illustrative ones will be reviewed here. HIV infection is addressed because of its increasing prevalence, and hyperthyroidism because of its clinical frequency. Hypoglycemia, although controversial, is an important syndrome for clinicians to understand because many patients correctly or incorrectly self-diagnose this disorder. Pheochromocytoma, finally, is a rare disorder but one with important lessons for the clinician seeking to understand anxiety disorders.

Human Immunodeficiency Virus

The HIV virus is estimated to have already infected 13 million people worldwide ("AIDS: The Third Wave," *Lancet* 1994), including approximately 1.5 million Americans. Ten percent of all patients with AIDS will initially present with CNS symptoms. Furthermore, 40%–60% of all patients with AIDS will manifest CNS symptoms at some point during their illness. At death and on autopsy, 80%–90% will have signs of neurological involvement (Fauci and Lane 1991). The anxiety that occurs in AIDS patients can stem from the neurological changes, the psychosocial stress of the disorder, or a combination of both factors.

Some HIV-seropositive patients appear to experience anxiety with or without cognitive defects. This anxiety is due primarily to organic disease and may be unaccompanied by other symptoms of organic illness (Atkinson et al. 1988; Bornstein et al. 1993; Grant et al. 1987; Ostrow 1987). In some anxious but otherwise "asymptomatic" AIDS patients, therefore, and in any individual with medical or lifestyle risks for HIV infection who presents with new emotional or behavioral symptoms, organic factors should be considered in the evaluation of the patient's problems (Grant et al. 1987).

Psychosocially induced anxiety, too, is understandably associated with AIDS and the danger of contracting AIDS. The worrying of low- or high-risk people about whether they or someone they know has contracted the disease has become a growing public health problem in itself. For those who are contemplating being tested or who are awaiting test results, anxiety can reach intolerable levels. Those who test positive for the HIV virus face an increased risk for subsequent anxiety, panic, depression, and suicide. In addition to primary HIV effects and opportunistic infections that can produce behavioral symptoms, many of the drugs used to treat AIDS and its complications can cause a spectrum of toxic effects that include anxiety symptoms. As the disease progresses, it can become increasingly difficult to distinguish whether associated anxiety is predominantly due to organic, psychosocial, or treatment-related factors (Perry et al. 1993). Frequently, a combination of causes is present.

As an additional complication, AIDS patients very often experience an increasing impairment in their quality of life as they undergo a progressive deterioration in their health. In New York City, 86% of the first 1,065 AIDS patients survived their initial hospitalization, but 46% of those survivors spent at least 30% of their remaining weeks or months in a hospital and 32% required hospitalization for at least half of their remaining lifetime (Dilley 1990). The AIDS patient must deal with a progressive and terminal illness, often loss of employment, possible social isolation, and potential financial difficulties. Any of these losses could produce marked anxiety of a psychosocially based etiology in AIDS sufferers. Psychotherapeutic focus on grieving, successful life adaption, and cautious use of psychotropic medications is believed by many clinicians to be helpful.

> Mr. B, a 51-year-old married man with two children in college, was a professor at a local university and a deacon in his church. He was also conflicted about his sexual orientation. Over the course of his 26-year marriage, he had had numerous and anonymous sexual encounters with men. In his psychotherapy, he explored his sexual ambivalence and his guilt in hiding it from his wife and children. Mr. B's feelings of anxiety and shame hampered his effectiveness at work and hindered intimacy at home. The thoughts and discussions related to HIV

testing were extremely anxiety-provoking to him and he feared that he would commit suicide if he were to test positive. He attributed his recent (2 months' duration) fatigue, increased anxiety, and weight loss to his fear of the HIV test. Once he obtained the HIV test, which was positive, he exhibited panic attacks and depression. He felt he could not tell his wife, and he continued to engage in unprotected sex with her, albeit with diminished frequency. When finally Mr. B agreed to tell his wife, however, he told her he had contracted the infection from female prostitutes. Mrs. B tested negative. Mr. B developed increased anxiety and slight paranoid ideation. He eventually acquired encephalitis secondary to cytomegalovirus (CMV). Although a definitive etiological diagnosis of Mr. B's anxiety was never reached, his symptoms were partially relieved by supportive psychotherapy with adjunctive pharmacotherapy. Clonazepam was used to target his anxiety symptoms, and haloperidol in low doses relieved the paranoid ideation.

Hyperthyroidism

Hyperthyroidism is a relatively common illness, affecting approximately 2% of women and 0.2% of men (Larsen 1992). It is usually diagnosed by clinical history, physical examination, and measurement of serum T4 and the thyroid hormone–binding ratio (free thyroxine index [FTI]). Hyperthyroidism most often affects adults between the ages of 20 and 50 years. As the body responds to an excess of thyroid hormone, several physiological symptoms become evident. These include tremor, sweating, heat intolerance, tachycardia, palpitations, anorexia, and even peptic ulcers.

Other behavioral manifestations of this syndrome include anxiety, nervousness, rapid speech, and emotional lability (Larsen 1992). When the onset of hyperthyroidism is rapid, its symptoms can be confused with nonorganic anxiety and falsely attributed to situational factors. Comorbid substance abuse or the effects of prescribed medications on primary anxiety can also obscure the diagnosis (American Psychiatric Association 1994).

Treatment of hyperthyroidism usually involves addressing the underlying disease of the thyroid and may necessitate surgery, radiation, and/or hormone replacement therapy. Even after treatment and correction of the underlying hormone imbalance, anxiety may persist. This subsequent anxiety often responds to conventional antianxiety medication (Nemiah 1985). Exogenous thyroid hormone, prescribed for the treatment of hypothyroidism or to augment antidepressant treatment, can also produce symptoms of anxiety in some individuals at therapeutic doses and in many when taken in excessive amounts.

> Ms. C, a 34-year-old woman diagnosed with a mixed personality disorder, had been steadily employed as a paralegal. She had been in psychotherapy for 1 year. During that time, she began to have increasing difficulties with both her job and her boyfriend. As she sensed both areas of functioning to be deteriorating, she experienced mounting anxiety. Ms. C was given the diagnosis of adjustment disorder with anxious mood and was started on clonazepam 0.5 mg twice a day. This proved helpful. Over the next 3 months, her anxiety symptoms necessitated a gradual increase of clonazepam up to 1.0 mg five times a day. At this point, Ms. C complained of feeling both anxious and chronically fatigued.
>
> Basic blood measurements were ordered, including a thyroid screen. The results showed hyperthyroidism. Ms. C was referred to an endocrinologist, who diagnosed a toxic multinodular goiter. Although this was treated successfully with surgery, Ms. C's anxiety remained, and again she was treated with clonazepam 0.5 mg, twice a day, with success. After 2 months, the clonazepam was discontinued. In retrospect, it was apparent that Ms. C's gradually increasing symptoms of hyperthyroidism were combined with or perhaps even mistaken for primary anxiety.

Hypoglycemia

Hypoglycemia is a nonspecific pathophysiological state like fever or pain rather than a disease in itself. It is diagnosed when the blood glucose level, normally above 60 mg/dl, is determined to be below 45 mg/dl. The physical manifestations commonly attributed to hypoglycemia include tremor, sweating, hunger, and dizziness. Causes of this condition include diabetes, ethanol abuse, pancreatic cancer, and a variety of endocrine disorders—for example, adrenocortical insufficiency, hypopituitarism, and growth hormone deficiency (Service 1992).

The varied psychiatric symptoms alleged to accompany hypoglycemia include subjective anxiety, irritability, shakiness, palpitations, and abnormal behavior (Service 1992). In severe hypoglycemia, depression or fatigue can ensue. Blood glucose levels that persist below 20 mg/dl for a protracted period of time can result in brain damage or dementia that may not be reversible by subsequent correction of the glucose level.

A potentially misleading aspect of hypoglycemia is that acute episodes can resemble ethanol intoxication. In both conditions, gait can be unsteady and speech slurred. The bizarre, delirious behavior sometimes associated with low glucose levels can divert attention from consideration of somatic diagnoses. In addition, a hypoglycemic person's breath can have an ethanol-like odor, because the body burns fat and proteins, producing aldehydes. Treatment must address the underlying physical disturbance.

Functional hypoglycemia is sometimes diagnosed when no specific etiology can be identified. In this condition, an overactive pancreas is hypothesized, producing hormones that cause the blood sugar to fall to symptomatic levels within 2–4 hours after eating. Functional hypoglycemia is a controversial diagnosis. Many in the medical field feel that the condition is overdiagnosed in patients with problems that are primarily psychogenic. Although functional hypoglycemia has no known cure, dietary intervention is considered by some proponents of this diagnostic syndrome to be the most beneficial intervention. One suggested diet encourages high protein and low carbohydrate intake, a regimen thought to promote a more steady glucose level (Service 1992).

Ms. D, a 25-year-old married woman, complained of both

anxiety and fatigue. She described morning exhaustion and discrete episodes of anxiety throughout the day. She denied any drug or ethanol use and was taking no medications. Previous internists had diagnosed fibromyalgia and chronic fatigue syndrome; they had also noted Ms. D's tendency to somatize conflicts and considered her a hypochondriac.

Her current internist questioned her previous diagnoses and performed a 2-hour postprandial glucose test. Ms. D was found to be hypoglycemic. Her anxiety and chronic fatigue improved with dietary intervention. With a high-protein and low-carbohydrate diet, Ms. D was better able to maintain a steady glucose level.

Pheochromocytoma

Pheochromocytoma is a rare adrenocortical tumor that secretes catecholamines and affects about one of every 1,000 hypertensive patients (Cryer 1992). Its description illustrates how even uncommon and episodic illnesses should be considered in the differential diagnosis of anxiety disorders.

This disease primarily occurs in adults and affects males and females equally. Initially pheochromocytoma presents with episodic hypertension and intense anxiety or paniclike symptoms. Over time, 60% of patients will develop constant hypertension and anxiety (Nemiah 1985). It is the remaining 40%, those who continue to experience episodic hypertension and anxiety, who can be mistakenly treated for generalized anxiety or panic disorder.

The diagnosis of pheochromocytoma is made by a 24-hour urine assay that shows elevated quantities of catecholamines or catecholamine metabolites. The diagnosis can often be made with one urine collection, provided that the patient is symptomatic at the time of the sampling. Treatment usually involves surgical removal of the tumor except in cases where the tumor is too far advanced or is highly malignant with metastasis. Prognosis is often good, with an overall 95% survival at 5 years; however, the malignant variety has a poorer prognosis of only 50% survival at 5 years. The hypertension resolves completely in 75% of cases once the tumor is removed. In the remaining 25%, the hypertension is usually controllable with antihypertensive drugs. The panic or anxiety is also thought to abate with the tumor's removal, although in some cases the panic remains. It is then usually responsive to conventional antipanic medication (Landsberg and Young 1991).

> Mr. E, a 29-year-old man, was a successful stockbroker. He had a history of ethanol and cocaine abuse but had been sober for approximately 1 year prior to evaluation. He credited his successful sobriety to three factors: psychotherapy, Narcotics Anonymous, and the onset of panic attacks while using cocaine. Although Mr. E's job and personal life had improved with sobriety and psychotherapy, his panic attacks continued. He had been treated with both TCAs and long-acting benzodiazepines, with inconsistent success. His internist measured blood chemistries and obtained an ECG but found no abnormalities. Eventually, Mr. E was found to have intermittent hypertension and a 24-hour urine catecholamine test was suggested. A pheochromocytoma was revealed. Mr. E was treated successfully with medication and surgery. In retrospect, it was easy to see how his panic attacks were mistakenly attributed to cocaine and ethanol abuse. There was nearly a 2-year delay from initiation of symptoms to diagnosis of pheochromocytoma. The presence of a more common disorder, the rarity of pheochromocytoma, and the episodic nature of its symptoms fooled both his therapist and his internist. Mr. E's incomplete response to antipanic medication and the finding of hypertension resulted in a more extensive medical workup.

■ Conclusions

Anxiety, whether from a primarily psychosocial or organic etiology, is characterized by a nonspecific cluster of signs and symptoms. Even when anxiety is psychosocial in origin, comorbid substance abuse or medical complications can confuse the processes of diagnosis and treatment. In addition, many laboratory tests can yield incomplete or inconclusive results. A basic understanding of autonomic function, a thorough medical and psychiatric history, and appropriate physical examination and laboratory testing are valuable tools in determining the factors that contribute to a patient's anxiety. The psychotherapist is advised to consider the value of such a comprehensive assessment at the onset of treatment for anxiety or at a later stage if response to treatment has been less than anticipated.

▌ References

AIDS: the third wave (editorial). Lancet 343:186–188, 1994

Altamura AC, Montgomery SA, Wernicke JF: The evidence for 20 mg/day of fluoxetine as the optimal dose in the treatment of depression. Br J Psychiatry 153:109–112, 1988

American Psychiatric Association, Diagnostic and Statistical Manual of Mental Disorders, 4th Edition. Washington, DC, American Psychiatric Association, 1994

Aniline O, Pitts FN: Phencyclidine (PCP): a review and perspectives. Crit Rev Toxicol 10:145–177, 1982

Atkinson JH, Grant I, Kennedy CJ, et al: Prevalence of psychiatric disorders among men infected with human immunodeficiency virus. Arch Gen Psychiatry 45:859–864, 1988

Berkow R: The Merck Manual. Rahway, NJ, Merck Research Laboratories, 1992

Bornstein RA, Pace P, Rosenberger P, et al: Depression and neuropsychological performance in asymptomatic HIV infection. Am J Psychiatry 150:922–926, 1993

Breslau N, Kilbey M, Andreski P: Vulnerability to psychopathology in nicotine-dependent smokers: an epidemiologic study of young adults. Am J Psychiatry 150:941–946, 1993

Charney DS, Heninger GR, Jatlow PI: Increased anxiogenic effects of caffeine in panic disorders. Arch Gen Psychiatry 42:233–243, 1985

Clemeatz GL, Dailey JW: Psychotropic effects of caffeine. Am Fam Physician 37:167–172, 1988

Crack. Medical Letter 28:69–70, 1986

Cryer PS: The adrenal medullae, in Cecil Textbook of Medicine, 19th Edition. Edited by Wyngaarden J, Smith L, Bennett J. Philadelphia, PA, WB Saunders, 1992, pp 1390–1396

Diamond I: Alcoholism and alcohol abuse, in Cecil Textbook of Medicine, 19th Edition. Edited by Wyngaarden JB, Smith LH, Bennett JC. Philadelphia, PA, WB Saunders, 1992, pp 44–47

Dilley J: Psychosocial impact of AIDS: overview, in The AIDS Knowledge Base. Edited by Cohen P, Sande M, Volberding P. Waltham, MA, Medical Publishing Group, 1990, pp 5.13.1-1–5.13.1-3

Dilsaver SC, Kronfol Z, Sackellares JC, et al: Antidepressant withdrawal syndromes: evidence supporting the cholinergic overdrive hypothesis. J Clin Psychopharmacol 3:157–164, 1983

Durant RH, Rickert VI, Ashworth CS, et al: Use of multiple drugs among adolescents who use anabolic steroids. N Engl J Med 328:922–926, 1993

Ellis J: Is New York "a civilization slipping away"? Boston Globe, September 13, 1993, p 11A

Fauci AS, Lane HC: The acquired immunodeficiency syndrome (AIDS), in Harrison's Principles of Internal Medicine. Edited by Wilson JD, Braunwald E, Isselbacher KJ, et al. New York, McGraw-Hill, 1991, pp 1402–1410

Gawin FH, Ellinwood EH: Cocaine and other stimulants. N Engl J Med 318:1173–1182, 1988

Glassman A: Cigarette smoking: implications for psychiatric illness. Am J Psychiatry 150:546–553, 1993

Grant I, Atkinson JH, Hesselink JR, et al: Evidence for early central nervous system involvement in the acquired immunodeficiency syndrome (AIDS) and other human immunodeficiency virus (HIV) infections. Ann Intern Med 107:828-836, 1987

Haddad LM, Roberts JR: A general approach to the emergency management of poisoning, in Poisoning and Drug Overdose, 2nd Edition. Edited by Haddad LM, Roberts JR. Philadelphia, PA, Harcourt, Brace, & Jovanovich, 1990, pp 2–22

Haynes RC: Adrenocorticotropic hormone: adrenocortical steroids and their synthetic analogs, in Goodman and Gilman's The Pharmacological Basis of Therapeutics, 8th Edition. Edited by Gilman A, Rall TW, Nies AS, et al. New York, Pergamon, 1990, pp 1431–1462

Henry JA, Jeffreys KJ, Dawling S: Toxicity and deaths from 3,4-methylenedioxymethamphetamine ("ecstasy"). Lancet 340:384–387, 1992

Higgins S, Delaney D, Budney A, et al: A behavioral approach to achieving initial cocaine abstinence. Am J Psychiatry 148:1218–1224, 1991

Hoffman B, Lefkowitz FJ: Catecholamines and sympathomimetic drugs, in Goodman and Gilman's The Pharmacological Basis of Therapeutics, 8th Edition. Edited by Gilman A, Rall TW, Nies AS. New York, Pergamon, 1990, pp 187–220

Holbrook J, Aghababian R: The alcoholic patient, in Emergency Medicine, 2nd Edition. Edited by May HL, Aghababian RV, Fleisher GR, et al. Boston, Little, Brown, 1992, pp 2021–2026

Hoyt DW, Finnigan RE, Nee T, et al: Drug testing in the workplace: are methods legally defensible? JAMA 258:504–509, 1987

Iserson KV: Caffeine and nicotine, in Poisoning and Drug Overdose. Edited by Haddad LM, Winchester JF. Philadelphia, PA, WB Saunders, 1990, pp 867–876

Ishak KS: Hepatic neoplasms associated with contraceptive and anabolic steroids. Recent Results Cancer Res 66:73–128, 1979

Jaffe JH: Drug addiction and drug abuse, in Goodman and Gilman's The Pharmacological Basis of Therapeutics, 8th Edition. Edited by Gilman A, Rall TW, Nies AS. New York, Pergamon, 1990, pp 522–573

Jaffe JH, Martin WR: Opioid analgesics and antagonists, in Goodman and Gilman's The Pharmacological Basis of Therapeutics, 8th Edition. Edited by Gilman A, Rall TW, Nies AS. New York, Pergamon, 1990, pp 485–521

Khantzian EJ: The self-medication hypothesis of addictive disorders: focus on heroin and cocaine dependence. Am J Psychiatry 142:1259–1264, 1985

Kong D: On toll of alcohol versus drugs, even the experts don't agree. Boston Globe, January 30, 1990, pp 1, 10

Koranyi EK: Morbidity and rate of undiagnosed physical illnesses in a psychiatric clinic population. Arch Gen Psychiatry 36:414–419, 1979

Landsberg L, Young JB: Pheochromocytoma, in Harrison's Principles of Internal Medicine. Edited by Wilson JD, Braunwald E, Isselbacher KJ, et al. New York, McGraw-Hill, 1991, pp 1735–1739

Larsen PR: The thyroid, in Cecil Textbook of Medicine, 19th Edition. Edited by Wyngaarden J, Smith L, Bennett J. Philadelphia, PA, WB Saunders, 1992, pp 1248–1271

Lefkowitz RJ, Hoffman BB, Taylor P: Neurohumoral transmission: the autonomic and somatic motor nervous systems, in Goodman and Gilman's The Pharmacological Basis of Therapeutics, 8th Edition. Edited by Gilman A, Rall TW, Nies AS. New York, Pergamon, 1990, pp 84–121

Massion A, Warshaw M, Keller M: Quality of life and psychiatric morbidity in panic disorder and generalized anxiety disorder. Am J Psychiatry 150:600–607, 1993

McLellan AT, Woody GE, O'Brien CP: Development of psychiatric illness in drug abusers: role of drug preference. N Engl J Med 301:1310–1314, 1979

Miller LG, Jankovic J: Drug-induced dyskinesias, in Current Neurology, Vol 10. Edited by Appel SH. Chicago, IL, Year Book Medical, 1990, pp 321–355

Myers JK, Weissman MM, Tischler GL, et al: Six-month prevalence of psychiatric disorders in three communities, 1980 to 1982. Arch Gen Psychiatry 41:959–967, 1984

Nemiah J: Anxiety states, in Comprehensive Textbook of Psychiatry, 4th Edition. Edited by Kaplan H, Sadock B. Baltimore, MD, Williams & Wilkins, 1985, pp 891–894

Ostrow DG: Psychiatric consequences of AIDS: an overview. Int J Neurosci 32:669–676, 1987

Perry S, Jacobsberg L, Card C, et al: Severity of psychiatric symptoms after HIV testing. Am J Psychiatry 150:775–779, 1993

Pollack MH, Rosenbaum JF: Management of antidepressant-induced side effects: a practical guide for the clinician. J Clin Psychiatry 48:3–8, 1987

Rall TW: Drugs used in the treatment of asthma: the methylxanthines, cromolyn sodium and other agents, in Goodman and Gilman's The Pharmacological Basis of Therapeutics, 8th Edition. Edited by Gilman A, Rall TW, Nies AS. New York, Pergamon, 1990, pp 618–637

Rosenbaum JF, Woods SW, Groves JE, et al: Emergence of hostility during alprazolam treatment. Am J Psychiatry 141:792–793, 1984

Saklad SR: Overview of anxiety. Medicine and Psychiatry 2:1, 1985

Service FJ: Hypoglycemic disorders, in Cecil Textbook of Medicine, 19th Edition. Edited by Wyngaarden J, Smith L, Bennett J. Philadelphia, PA, WB Saunders, 1992, pp 1310–1317

Su T-P, Pagliaro M, Schmidt PJ, et al: Neuropsychiatric effects of anabolic steroids in male normal volunteers. JAMA 269:2760–2764, 1993

Syed IB: The effects of caffeine. Journal of the American Pharmaceutical Association 16:568, 1976

Weissman MM, Klerman GL, Markowitz JS, et al: Suicidal ideation and suicide attempts in panic disorder and attacks. N Engl J Med 321:1204–1214, 1984

The Anxious Substance Abuser
and the Anxious Clinician

Henry David Abraham, M.D.

F ew problems in psychiatry are more vexatious than those posed by substance-abusing patients who carry additional Axis I diagnoses. The clinical complexity of these patients is increasingly being noted in the literature (Brown and Barlow 1992; Galanter et al. 1994; Regier et al. 1990; Schuckit and Hesselbrock 1994). Comorbid substance use and other mental disorders are found in two-thirds of the homeless and in an equally large proportion of inpatients in inner-city general hospitals. The term *dually diagnosed,* now applied to such patients, is an unfortunate success story: unfortunate because the term is borrowed from the disci-

This work was supported by U.S. Public Health Service Grant RO1 DA07120-01A2.

275

pline of developmental disabilities, which has traditionally used it to refer to persons with mental retardation and additional psychopathology, and successful because the term appears nevertheless to be gaining wider use in the professional community. Although such dually diagnosed patients are receiving increasing attention from researchers (Cloninger et al. 1990; Landry et al. 1991), the treatment dilemma they present has no easy answers. While instinct urges ministering to a patient's depression, anxiety, or psychosis with a variety of pharmacotherapeutic tools, the possibility of an exacerbated addiction often stays the clinician's hand. The net result is either avoidance of the use of needed medication—leaving the patient untreated—or use of medication that may inadvertently contribute to the patient's abuse problem. This dilemma occurs particularly in the treatment of anxiety disorders associated with substance abuse, because the class of agents most commonly used for this purpose—the benzodiazepines—is abusable, addictive, and marketable by desperate addicted individuals in search of stronger fare.

The association of substance abuse with an anxiety disorder occurs at a higher-than-random rate. The Epidemiologic Catchment Area (ECA) program of the National Institute of Mental Health reported that, among 20,291 persons interviewed for mental disorders, 23.7% of those with a lifetime history of anxiety disorder also had a substance use disorder (Regier et al. 1990). Thirty-five and eight-tenths percent of individuals with panic disorder and 32.8% of those with obsessive-compulsive disorder carried a past or present diagnosis of substance abuse as well. In the Washington University Clinic study, 500 outpatients of the clinic were twice assessed with the same diagnostic instrument: once at the beginning of the study and again 6–12 years later (Cloninger et al. 1985). The data showed that both primary alcoholism and anxiety disorders were associated with secondary diagnoses over time. Cloninger (1987) found generalized anxiety disorder (GAD) to be associated with Type 1 alcohol dependence (characterized by onset after age 25, high risk-avoidance, infrequent antisocial behavior, loss of control of drinking, and guilt over drinking, among other variables). In contrast, somatization disorder was related to

Type 2 alcoholism (onset before age 25, low harm-avoidance, frequent antisocial behavior, and infrequent guilt about drinking). Cox and colleagues (1990) reviewed comorbidity in both anxiety disorder patients and alcoholic patients, and reported that 10%–20% of the former abused drugs, whereas 10%–40% of the latter reported panic-related anxiety. Van Ameringen et al. (1991), in a survey of 57 patients with social phobia, found that 28.1% of the sample were alcoholic and 15.8% were drug abusers.

Approaching the estimation of comorbidity from the other direction, Mirin and colleagues (1991) surveyed 350 patients on a substance abuse treatment unit for other psychiatric disorders. Thirty-seven percent of these substance abusers had additional Axis I diagnoses. Cocaine appeared to be associated with cyclothymia, and sedative-hypnotic abuse with GAD. In my study of 67 patients with post-LSD perceptual disorder, 29.5% had panic disorder, 3.8% had GAD, and 29.5% had both anxiety disorders in addition to hallucinogen-related perceptual disorder (H. D. Abraham, unpublished data, January 1995). A comparison with drug abusers without post-LSD perceptual disorder showed similar rates of GAD with or without panic, but the LSD perceptual disorder group had higher rates of panic disorder (57.8% compared with 38.8%, $P < .03$). The presence of panic disorder is associated with an elevated risk for suicidal behavior, and Lepine and colleagues (1993) demonstrated a further increase in this risk in the presence of concurrent substance abuse.

▌ The Chicken or the Egg

No longer of strictly academic interest in psychiatry, the issue of temporal sequence in the association of anxiety and substance use disorders is likely to have a decisive impact on clinical diagnoses, treatment choices, and outcomes, simply because treatment of primary disorders can often favorably affect the prognoses or treatments of secondary ones. It has been proposed, for example, that social phobia patients develop alcoholism secondarily, from attempts at self-medication (Kushner et al. 1990). This proposal suggests that aggressive treatment of social phobia could prevent later alcohol abuse, an important but untested idea (Cox et al. 1990). The self-medication hypothesis of alcohol abuse, on the other hand, is not likely to be universally applicable to all alcoholic persons with anxiety disorders. There are patients whose anxiety is fed by an interminable cycle of alcohol abuse and withdrawal, and those whose use of alcohol may represent self-medication for a chronic anxiety disorder. The anxiety of an alcoholic patient who cycles in and out of withdrawal before seeking medical attention may appear indistinguishable from that of a patient with intermittently symptomatic primary GAD. Similar diagnostic confusion can occur with anxious abusers of psychostimulants such as cocaine, amphetamines, hallucinogens (e.g., LSD), and cannabis, and, of course, with persons withdrawing from sedative-hypnotics. In the association of drug abuse with anxiety, a crucial question is which condition came first in a given patient's life. Although documenting an order of onset between substance use and anxiety disorders is admittedly difficult and even at times impossible, success in that regard increases the likelihood that a helpful therapeutic strategy will be instituted and a potentially harmful one avoided.

Co-occurrence of panic disorder and substance abuse may assume several possible patterns: panic disorder may lead to substance abuse; drug abuse may lead to panic; each disorder may arise independently or in response to a common proximate cause; or the two disorders may arise independently but interact with one another to exacerbate the clinical situation. Furthermore, the relationship between anxiety and substance abuse is a complex one that depends on the interaction of factors such as drug type, preexisting psychopathology, effects of drug use and withdrawal, intrapsychic and intrafamilial conflicts, and the natural histories of both conditions (Meyer and Kranzler 1990). Although order-of-onset studies in anxiety and substance abuse may often be compromised by such confounding factors, they nevertheless begin to address the critical issues of causality in the dually diagnosed patient.

■ Studies of Order of Onset in Patients With Both Anxiety and Substance Use Disorders

Although proof of causality in psychiatry is rarely achieved, approaches to the problem of anxiety disorders and substance abuse have yielded interesting findings. What follows is a brief review of temporal associations between anxiety and substance use disorders.

Alcohol and Anxiety Disorders

The majority of drug abuse studies available on comorbidity focus on alcoholism. Although the association between alcoholism and anxiety is clinically recognized, it is not established whether one causes the other or the two occur independently. Meyer and Kranzler (1990) posited that simple models of cause and effect may not adequately address the heterogeneity of alcoholism.

Alcohol, traditionally, is considered to oppose anxiety, yet anxiety is a component of alcohol withdrawal. In samples of alcoholic patients, the prevalence of anxiety has varied from 10% to 44% (Bowen et al. 1984; Hesselbrock et al. 1985). Conversely, 13% of 254 agoraphobic individuals in one study had alcoholism, and one-third of these alcoholic agoraphobia patients acknowledged using alcohol to control their anxiety symptoms (Bibb and Chambless 1986).

Kushner and colleagues (1990) reviewed 15 studies of comorbid alcohol and anxiety disorders. Study groups came from both alcoholic and anxiety disorder populations. In 11 studies, alcohol abuse tended to follow agoraphobia and social phobia as a consequence of self-medication. In 3 studies, panic disorder appeared equally likely to occur before or after alcoholism, and in 1 study, GAD appeared to follow pathological drinking. Another study (Starcevic et al. 1993) examined 54 patients with panic disorder and other comorbid conditions and found that those who abused alcohol and drugs prior to the onset of panic tended to have experienced the onset of panic closer to the onset of drug and alcohol abuse than to the onset of other comorbid disorders. This finding suggested to the investigators that drug use may have played a causal role in panic disorder.

The linkage between alcoholism and anxiety disorders may have a genetic component. Evidence supporting this premise has been generated by studies that measured the prevalence rate for one of these disorders among biological relatives (e.g., monozygotic and dizygotic twins, first-degree relatives) of individuals affected with the other disorder. Leckman and colleagues (1983), for example, found the prevalence of alcoholism to be higher than expected in relatives of patients with major depression and panic disorder. It is anticipated that current efforts to identify alleles associated with alcoholism and the anxiety disorders will eventually illuminate the mechanism of comorbidity.

Psychostimulant Drugs and Panic Attacks

Anxiety symptoms have long been associated with the use of psychostimulant drugs such as caffeine, amphetamines, and cocaine (Snyder 1972). In a sample of 85 cocaine users, chronic effects of cocaine included anxiety symptoms in 44% (Siegel 1977). In 1986, Aronson and Craig described three cases of panic disorder that was precipitated by recreational use of intranasal cocaine and that continued to occur autonomously. Rosenbaum (1986) reported on a patient with a positive family history for panic attacks whose own panic attacks appeared to be precipitated by a single night's ingestion of a gram of cocaine. He suggested that stimulants such as cocaine might lower the threshold of limbic arousal chronically, thereby setting the stage for multiple attacks. Pohl and colleagues (1987) subsequently described a patient whose panic disorder followed the abuse of amphetamines and cocaine. The patient's first attack occurred while snorting "over 1 gram" of cocaine. It was followed by frequent panic attacks not associated with the use of psychostimulant drugs.

In 1989, Louie and colleagues described 10 patients who developed chronic panic attacks after substantial cocaine use. The fact that only 1 of the 10 patients studied had a first-degree relative with panic disorder suggested that the disorder was acquired rather than primary. These patients' symptoms were explained by Louie et al. as arising from limbic-neuronal hyperexcitability induced by cocaine kindling.

Abraham (1989) employed computational electroencephalogram (EEG) techniques to provide the first evidence supporting this kindling theory: a finding of abnormal electrophysiology in 15 panic patients with substance abuse. A larger group of 50 patients with panic disorder and/or substance abuse (Abraham and Duffy 1991) was divided into subgroups of uncomplicated panic, uncomplicated drug abuse/dependence, and dually diagnosed drug abuse and panic patients. Quantitative EEG (qEEG) revealed nondominant temporal abnormalities in the panic cases and bitemporal abnormalities in the dual-diagnosis group. These findings were consistent with previously published findings from positron-emission tomography (PET) scan (Reiman et al. 1984) and magnetic resonance imaging (MRI) studies (Fontaine et al. 1990) in panic patients. No significant abnormalities emerged in the uncomplicated drug abuse/dependence group. Post hoc comparisons between the pure and the dually diagnosed drug abusers revealed that 92.9% of the latter had used psychostimulants, compared with 36.8% of the former. Of the panic patients with cocaine histories, 86% reported that drug use had preceded their first lifetime occurrence of panic.

Ellinwood and Kilbey (1980) have conceptualized psychomotor stimulant–induced behavior as attributable to conditioning, kindling, metabolic adaptations to a drug, decreases in neurotransmitters such as dopamine, and increased numbers of dopamine receptors. It is believed that these processes take place at least in part within the limbic system, an interconnected ring of neural structures communicating between the higher cortical centers and the hypothalamus and related by Papez (1937) to the modulation of emotion. Cocaine directly alters electrophysiological function in the limbic system (Dafny et al. 1979; Lesse and Collins 1979, 1980). An effort to replicate the qEEG abnormalities in subjects with comorbid cocaine abuse/dependence and panic disorder is currently under way in Abraham's research group.

Cannabis and Panic Attacks

Panic reactions to cannabis are considered the commonest adverse effect of this drug (Thomas 1993). Data supporting this assertion have derived from case histories, retrospective surveys of drug users, and experimental administrations of the drug. Bromberg (1939), for example, reported 14 cases of acute panic secondary to the experimental administration of marijuana. Although adverse reactions to cannabis may occupy points along a spectrum from dysphoria to panic, such reactions are only occasionally severe enough to require clinical attention (Abraham 1984).

LSD and Panic Disorder

As previously noted, Abraham (unpublished data, January 1995) has found higher rates of panic disorder both with and without concurrent GAD among post-LSD perceptual disorder patients than among drug and alcohol abusers without post-LSD perceptual disorder. Studies of temporal sequencing remain to be done for this population.

Sedatives and Generalized Anxiety Disorder

Interestingly, in women a history of an anxiety disorder combined with depression increases the likelihood of using prescribed anxiolytics significantly more than does a history of an anxiety disorder alone (Pariente et al. 1992). This finding raises questions about the interrelationships of anxiolytic therapy with anxiety and depression and emphasizes the potential value of order-of-onset studies that would elucidate these relationships. Unfortunately, no such studies are yet available.

▌ Treatment of the Dually Diagnosed Patient

The treatment approach outlined in the following subsections is applicable to any patient with both substance abuse and another psychiatric disorder. It prioritizes the need for accurate diagnosis and on this basis divides treatment into three phases. During the acute phase of treatment, it is common for either concurrent diagnoses or drug toxicity and withdrawal symptoms to confound one another. During the subacute phase, early sobriety may begin to yield evidence of concurrent diagnoses, the relative order of onset of comorbid conditions, and the therapeutic approaches most likely to be successful. During the chronic phase, the goals are the stable maintenance of therapeutic gains and attention to relapse prevention.

Acute Phase

The goals of treatment in the acute phase are listed in Table 9–1. Of the multiple agents commonly abused, it is withdrawal from alcohol or the hypnosedatives that carries the highest morbidity and mortality.

The treatment of alcohol withdrawal has been thoroughly reviewed elsewhere (Schuckit 1987). A guideline for the treatment of alcohol withdrawal in use at our program is detailed in Table 9–2.

There is no substitute for timely diagnosis and intervention in alcohol withdrawal, because symptoms escalate rapidly to dangerous levels when left untreated. Approximately 5% of alcoholic patients develop severe withdrawal symptoms, including confusion, hallucinations, delusions, agitation, and seizures. The mortality rate of untreated alcohol withdrawal approaches 5%. Physical examination of the individual undergoing withdrawal from alcohol should focus on those organ systems most affected by alcohol—namely, the central nervous system (CNS), the liver and gastrointestinal tract, and the cardiovascular system. In addition, metabolic regulation of glucose and electrolytes may show evidence of dysfunction. While mild or even moderate alcohol withdrawal may be treated in an outpatient setting, severe withdrawal is an indication for admission to an intensive care setting. Patients with moderate withdrawal symptoms, too, may require intensive care when other medical complications are present, such as trauma, infection, gastrointestinal bleeding, or congestive heart failure. Benzodiazepines are the treatment of choice for acute withdrawal symptoms, although psychotic individuals may require neuroleptics adjunctively. Intravenous benzodiazepines have been associated with respiratory arrest and should be administered only in settings in which resuscitation services are available. Parenteral benzodiazepines may be used when oral administration is impossible—for example, lorazepam at 2–4 mg intramuscularly every hour, or at 1–2 mg intravenously every 5–10 minutes, not to exceed 20 mg/hour or 50 mg/shift. Lorazepam and oxazepam, which are not metabolized by the liver, are the benzodiazepines of choice in the patient who has hepatic dysfunction. The patient's mental status must be monitored closely, especially when encephalopathy is present. Pharmacotherapy of acute and uncomplicated alcohol withdrawal seldom requires more than 3–5 days.

Table 9–1.   Goals for treating substance users with anxiety symptoms during the acute phase

---

1. Manage drug withdrawal symptoms.
2. Establish an early therapeutic contract.
3. Enroll significant others in treatment.
4. Avoid all anxiolytics other than for withdrawal of alcohol or sedative-hypnotics using established protocols.
5. Encourage early involvement with inspirational therapies.
6. Start systematic evaluation of lifetime history.
7. Review all lifetime records.
8. Conduct corroborative interviews with family member(s) for lifetime historical data.
9. Defer concurrent diagnoses for at least 1 month while observing symptom evolution.

Table 9–2.   Detoxification guidelines for alcohol withdrawal

---

Goals

1. To identify patients at risk for developing alcohol withdrawal
2. To assist in the planning and implementation of their *safe* and *aggressive* detoxification
3. To minimize the likelihood of potentially dangerous neurological complications of alcohol withdrawal, including agitation, seizures, delirium tremens, and/or death

Key points

1. While some patients at risk for alcohol withdrawal seek detoxification, others must be identified through appropriate clinical assessment.
2. When patients at risk for alcohol withdrawal are affected by medical illnesses or are concurrently dependent on other recreational drugs, their detoxification may require additional precautions to address the increased likelihood of medical complications.
3. The presence of alcohol intoxication or of a measurable blood alcohol concentration does not imply medical safety, because withdrawal symptoms reflect the presence of a decreasing rather than an absolute blood alcohol level.
4. The risk of potentially lethal alcohol withdrawal symptoms in an untreated patient can last up to 10 days. The concurrent abuse of benzodiazepines can further prolong the period of danger.

Routine orders

1. Each patient's assessment includes a *medical history* (including questions about substance abuse and other psychiatric disorders) and a *physical examination*. Particular attention is focused on the systems most susceptible to alcohol's destructive effects: the central nervous system, liver, gastrointestinal system, and heart. Mental status examination includes assessment of orientation, alertness, short-term memory, mood, hallucinations, delusions, and suicidality. The patient's hydration and nutritional status are also assessed.
2. *Laboratory studies* provide helpful data:
   a. A serum toxicology screen may be used to provide a measure of the blood alcohol level (BAL) and screen for the presence of some recreational drugs.
   b. A low hematocrit or positive test for stool occult blood may suggest the presence of gastrointestinal blood loss.

(continued)

Table 9–2.   Detoxification guidelines for alcohol withdrawal
(*continued*)

    c.   Liver dysfunction may be inferred from the presence of low serum albumin, elevated bilirubin, or coagulopathy.

    d.   Electrolytes, including magnesium (Mg^{++}), are measured in order to detect and plan treatment for potentially dangerous imbalances.

3.   Vitamins are given to replace deficient bodily supplies:

    a.   Thiamine 50–100 mg is given orally to reduce the risk of Wernicke's encephalopathy. This dosage is continued daily for 7 days.

    b.   A daily multivitamin supplement provides sufficient quantities of other vitamins.

4.   Benzodiazepines are the medications of choice in the detoxification of patients with uncomplicated alcohol withdrawal:

    a.   The first 72 hours following the last drink is a high-risk period for escalation of withdrawal symptoms. Benzodiazepines should be continued through this period with appropriate monitoring of mental status and vital signs.

    b.   Diazepam is one of several preferred benzodiazepines for detoxification because the long half-life of its active metabolite allows for a gradual waning of pharmacologic effect.

    c.   For mild to moderate uncomplicated alcohol withdrawal, administer diazepam 20 mg by mouth every 1–2 hours until a total of 60 mg is reached. Thereafter, administer 5- to 10-mg doses as needed every 1–2 hours for control of specified target symptoms. Total daily dose will not routinely exceed 75 mg. The presence of medical complications such as head trauma, pneumonia, active cardiopulmonary disease, significant gastrointestinal hemorrhage, significant pancreatitis, metabolic derangement, recurrent seizures, hepatic or renal failure, significant fluid depletion, or age greater than 50 suggest admission to an intensive care unit for closer monitoring.

    d.   For severe withdrawal, diazepam may be administered intravenously in injections of 5- to 10-mg doses. These should be given slowly, and resuscitation equipment should be available in the event of respiratory compromise. Total dosage will not routinely exceed 100 mg/hour or 250 mg/shift (8 hours). An intensive care unit is the preferred setting for this intervention.

Table 9–2.   Detoxification guidelines for alcohol withdrawal
             (continued)

---

   e.   A neuroleptic—for example, haloperidol—may be appropriate
        for use as one component of the treatment of withdrawal
        delirium associated with hyperarousal and agitation. Haloper-
        idol can also reduce associated psychotic symptoms. Haloper-
        idol and diazepam are synergistic in their sedative effects and
        relatively safe in combination. The use of haloperidol alone is
        discouraged because of potential lowering of the seizure
        threshold.

   f.   When haloperidol is used to treat psychotic symptoms with
        severe agitation, a recommended dose range is 0.5–2.0 mg
        administered intramuscularly or intravenously every 2 hours
        as needed, with close monitoring of vital signs and mental
        status and an upper limit of five doses in any 24-hour period.
        If psychotic symptoms and agitation persist beyond such treat-
        ment, it is appropriate to reassess the patient, considering
        alternative sources for these target symptoms.

5.   In mild, moderate, or severe withdrawal, symptoms are tracked
     with the Withdrawal Assessment Scale (Foy et al. 1988). Vital signs
     and behavioral status are assessed on a frequent basis.

6.   Early attention to the assessment and treatment of comorbid drug
     dependencies, medical illnesses, or psychosocial complications may
     facilitate discharge and reduce or defer relapse.

Source.   Adapted from Sandra Fitzgerald, M.D., and Anita Lewis, R.N.,
M.S., C.S., the Alcohol Treatment Resource Team, New England
Medical Center.

Withdrawal from alcohol and other addictive agents has traditionally been managed in inpatient settings, but with the cost of
medical care under increasing scrutiny by government and third-
party observers, financial support has been shifting from inpatient
treatment to outpatient detoxification programs. Thompson and
colleagues (1992), for example, analyzed data from 9,055 adult
intake interviews conducted over a 2½-year period in a managed
mental health care demonstration project. They found that assignments to hospitalization decreased during the first 6 months from

68% of substance abusers to 11% during the final period of the project. Thompson and co-workers further noted that such decisions appeared to be made as part of a policy to reduce all hospitalizations rather than simply the unneeded ones.

Although cost-cutting has value in the short run, the longer-range clinical outcomes of alternative forms of treatment may differ in ways that have not yet been identified. Controlled studies comparing inpatient with outpatient treatments have been compromised by a tendency for less-impaired patients to be assigned to outpatient treatment on a nonrandom basis (Collins 1993). Miller and Hester (1986), on the other hand, reviewed 26 controlled studies comparing inpatient with outpatient alcohol treatments. Each study used a random-assignment design. They found essentially no difference in outcome related to treatment site—in other words, treatment can be quite effective in either inpatient or outpatient settings. A similar finding was made by O'Brien and colleagues (1989); these authors reported significant improvements in patients dependent on both alcohol and cocaine who were treated with either partial or inpatient hospitalization.

Critical to the success of the earliest intervention efforts is the establishment of a therapeutic contract. Nothing helps this process more than an open, forthright discussion of the treatment program the patient is beginning. Minimizing surprises, maintaining consistency, defining limits, and respecting the patient's rights each contribute to the atmosphere of trust on which the treatment process depends. Ironically, a popular concept among clinicians treating dually diagnosed patients is that of *purposive behavior* (Jaffe 1990), which, if not an actual doctrine of distrust, at least requires the clinician to put trust on a back burner. Purposive behavior, a helpful concept to remember during interactions with a substance abuser, is the notion that more often than not, the "purpose" of any transaction between patient and clinician—despite the former's wish for recovery—is to obtain drugs. Drugs associated with such behavior include alcohol, sedative-hypnotics, cocaine, and stimulants. Purposive behaviors include any act imaginable whose aim is to procure drugs. The clinician's power to prescribe is not infrequently the preconscious or intended reason a substance abuser seeks help.

The countertransferences evoked in working with the addicted patient require fortitude in the clinician. It is not pleasant to believe or to come to the realization that one is being manipulated by someone who ostensibly is seeking help. In such situations, classical canons of medical ethics offer little to guide the clinician. What can be helpful, however, are a healthy skepticism of the patient's early self-appraisal, a sense of humor, an awareness of countertransference issues, an anticipation of manipulation, and clearly stated limits. Clinicians must also learn to resist the pressure to prescribe unneeded addictive agents to addicted individuals. And, ultimately, they must accept each patient's existential right to reject treatment, all the while remembering that it is also the patient's right to try again in the future. As regards this last point, Hippocrates' exhortation to do no harm is particularly apt, since substance abusers are among the few patients who may seek out mental health care in pursuit of goals antithetical to therapy. That being said, pharmacotherapy remains an appropriate treatment for overt alcohol or sedative-hypnotic withdrawal delirium, psychoses, or acutely suicidal states.

Additional help during the processes of diagnostic evaluation and therapeutic support often comes from persons who have intimate relationships with the patient. A spouse, significant other, or long-term friend may offer crucial data on needle habits or opportunistic infections in subjects at risk for human immunodeficiency virus (HIV)–related illness, or historical details about the development of anxiety and substance use disorders crucial to an understanding of order of onset.

One recommended aspect of the acute phase of treatment is a leisurely approach to diagnosis. The complex nature of most dual-diagnosis patients mandates a thoughtful and painstaking appraisal that is likely to extend well beyond the 1–2 hours of assessment that may suffice for diagnosing many other psychiatric conditions. It is valuable to initiate the process of obtaining records from all previously attended hospitals and clinics within the first day or so of admission into treatment. From these records, important information will be gleaned—regarding the patient's past drug use, withdrawal patterns, family supports, and so forth—that may not be available from the patient in the acute phase of treatment. A diagnostic period requiring weeks if not months may be necessary for elaborating a detailed understanding of the patient's biopsychosocial formulation. DSM-IV (American Psychiatric Association 1994) has addressed this problem by creating the category of *substance-induced anxiety disorder*. The availability of this diagnosis implies that substance-independent anxiety should be diagnosed only if symptoms persist at least 1 month beyond cessation of substance use.

Other factors associated with successful treatment include 1) inspirational therapies such as Alcoholics Anonymous (AA) or Narcotics Anonymous (NA), 2) substitute dependence (e.g., disulfiram), 3) a new love relationship, 4) willpower, 5) treatment in a drug clinic or hospital, and 6) adverse medical consequences of drug use (Vaillant 1983). Vaillant (1992), in addition, has shown, in a study of 100 heroin-addicted inmates, that prison and a year of parole resulted in abstinence at 1-year follow-up in 71% of the sample. For certain addictions dependent on illegal drug supplies, a "geographic cure" may be achieved by moving away from old drug contacts.

Psychotherapeutic experiences can play a central role in recovery from addiction, but exploratory therapy is not always the most appropriate approach. In a sobering report, Gerard and Saenger (1966) described an inverse relationship between exploratory psychotherapy and sobriety. "The less the clinic became involved in the intricacies of the determinants of the patient's symptoms, relationships, or defenses," they wrote of their experience with recovering alcoholics, "the more likely was the clinic to succeed in supporting change in drinking behavior" (p. 192). The beneficial role of inspirational group therapies, in contrast, is consistently reported even though such therapies have been sparsely researched. Among these groups, AA in particular has become widely known and appears to be quite helpful to those individuals able to maintain attendence. Half of AA's members drop out of the program within the first 3 months. Forty-one percent of those completing the first year will remain for a second year of membership. In a longitudinal study of 100 alcoholic patients over an 8-year period (Vaillant et al. 1983), attendance at AA was associated with social and clinical improvement.

Several obstacles, however, complicate the integration of AA with a comprehensive psychiatric approach. Many AA members are suspicious of—if not overtly hostile to—the use of psychotropic medications, an attitude underwritten in part by an awareness of the excessively casual prescribing practices of some physicians. Alcoholic individuals who take psychotropic medication are often criticized, in the no-nonsense language of AA, for "eating their booze." Physicians, in turn, have been skeptical of the "nonscientific" and quasi-religious AA philosophy, a group treatment model that historically has minimized the relevance of such complicating factors as comorbid psychiatric illnesses, prior religious preferences, educational level, and social class.

Thankfully, many individuals have worked to adapt AA to changing and special-needs constituencies, thereby increasing the program's accessibility and acceptability. In many urban areas, specialized AA meetings now address the needs of unique alcohol-abusing subpopulations such as homosexuals, clergy, cr physicians. Such gatherings are often referred to as "double trouble" AA groups. AA-based detoxification programs have become increasingly sensitive to the value of appropriately prescribed psychotropic medications, such as a manic alcoholic patient's lithium or a psychotic patient's neuroleptic.

A sensitive appraisal of a patient's religious and educational background helps to identify an appropriate program in which he or she can find support and healing. It is important for clinicians to be aware of their countertransference reactions regarding religiously oriented treatment and to remember the precept articulated by William James (1902/1985)—that "the treatment for dipsomania is religiomania" (p. 217). Even if more figuratively than literally true, this concept underscores the value of inspirational or religious support in the treatment of alcohol dependence. Finally, James also noted that General Booth, founder of the Salvation Army, considered that "the first vital step in saving outcasts consists in making them feel that some decent human being cares enough for them to take an interest in the question [of] whether they are to rise or sink" (James 1902/1985, p. 168). Such care is at the heart of successful early treatment of the addicted individual.

Subacute Phase

Following the first month of treatment, early sobriety is likely to permit identification of an individual's concurrent anxiety disorders. The concept of a month's delay in diagnosis is intended not as a mark chiseled in stone but rather as a helpful line in the sand. Clearly, diagnoses can be made before this time, but certainty in diagnosis is ultimately determined by the clarity and validity of each patient's clinical history, symptoms, and signs. During the first few days or weeks of sobriety, the diagnostic process is enshrouded in a mist of drug effects and drug-seeking behavior, which dissipates significantly as treatment ideals are internalized during the subsequent month.

The subacute treatment goals of early sobriety are itemized in Table 9–3. If the purpose of avoiding hasty diagnosis is to help direct treatment decisions for possible anxiety disorders, two other conditions are necessary before specific anxiolysis can be started: supplementation of a patient's report of symptoms with continuing, objective clinical observations consistent with an anxiety disorder diagnosis, and verification of sobriety through equally objective measures. In the office, anxiety may readily be observed through its manifestations of tachycardia, pallor, tremor, and perspiration. Objective signs of sobriety include reports from family members (except when family members are themselves substance-dependent), blood and urine screen results, and the absence of signs of drug toxicity such as slurred speech, contracted pupils, and the telltale smell of alcohol. When such conditions are met, therapeutic interventions targeted at an anxiety disorder diagnosis become more justifiable, and attribution of anxiety to drug toxicity or withdrawal becomes less compelling.

Therapy during the subacute phase becomes a process of selecting options from a continuum extending from the psychological and behavioral to the pharmacological. When pharmacotherapy is considered, an additional continuum extends from nonabusable to minimally abusable therapeutic agents. Simple phobias, for example, are appropriately treated with graded exposure, systematic desensitization, and other behavioral techniques, without recourse to medication (Foa and Kozak 1985). A patient with performance anxiety may be helped with a beta-adrenergic blocker effective for short intervals, such as during meetings or public presentations, thereby avoiding exposure to the risk associated with an abusable treatment agent (Brantigan et al. 1982). GAD may respond to dynamic or interpersonal psychotherapies, relaxation techniques (including self-hypnosis and meditation), or social therapy addressing a previously undisclosed conflict. Panic disorder, too, can be responsive to psychotherapeutic approaches (Craske 1988), although pharmacotherapy is very clearly a justifiable treatment option for this diagnosis (Klein et al. 1985).

When treating anxiety disorders in substance abuse patients, the process of choosing a medication is likely to assume more significance than is the case with other patients. This is not difficult

---

Table 9–3.   Subacute goals of treatment in early sobriety

Patient goals
1. Maintain sobriety.
2. Maintain ongoing patient-clinician contact.
3. Negotiate a therapeutic plan with the therapist.
4. Continue family, group, and inspirational therapies.
5. (Re)establish early healthy social contacts.

Clinician goals
1. Develop a preliminary diagnostic formulation of all Axis I disorders.
2. Negotiate with the patient regarding a treatment plan.
3. Initiate the first specific steps of anxiolysis.
4. Consolidate early treatment modalities.
5. Negotiate real and imagined conflicts between treatment modalities.
6. Document addictive behaviors.
7. Document ongoing anxiety symptoms and initial treatment responses.

to understand if one considers how many years addicted individuals may spend in acquiring drugs despite great risk, pain, illness, deprivation, shame, guilt, loss, crime, and abandonment. It is the hapless clinician indeed who steps onto this emotional minefield with closed eyes. Helpful in this situation are consistency, clarity, a prospective vision shared with the patient, and a painstaking degree of interpersonal honesty.

For most substance abusers with panic disorder, benzodiazepines (BZDs) are the drug class of last resort, if they are to be chosen at all. Indeed, substance abuse may be considered a relative contraindication for the use of BZDs. Comparable, and safer, results are likely to be achieved by treating the drug-abusing panic disorder patient with tricyclic antidepressants (TCAs) such as imipramine (Klein et al. 1985). For certain patients, the anticholinergic side-effect profile of dry mouth and blurred vision from TCAs may even generate an unexpected positive transference to treatment, since rare will be the patient who considers TCAs a placebo. Although less thoroughly researched, the selective serotonin reuptake inhibitors (SSRIs) are becoming popular agents for treating panic disorder (see Chapter 2). Buspirone, a nonaddictive serotonergic antianxiety agent that alleviates GAD and can sometimes play a role in the treatment of panic disorder, has an apparent advantage over BZDs in causing less significant tolerance and cognitive impairment. Unfortunately, this advantage is coupled with the drawback of a relatively delayed onset of antianxiety effect. In one study, buspirone's full effect required 12 weeks and was associated with a dropout rate of 73% (Tollefson et al. 1991).

Another class of nonaddictive agents that holds promise in treating the anxious person with an addiction is that of the beta-adrenergic blockers (see Chapter 1). Although few studies in drug-addicted populations are available, one double-blind, placebo-controlled trial among alcoholic inpatients showed significant anxiety reduction in response to 120 mg/day of propranolol (Gallant 1994).

An alternative approach relies upon the monoamine oxidase inhibitors (MAOIs), which were among the earliest agents shown to be effective against panic disorder (Sargant 1962). Close attention to compliance, drug habits, and diet are required, particularly in the patient given to abusing narcotics, cocaine, or stimulants, because these drugs have been associated with fatalities in patients concurrently taking MAOIs. Educating the patient regarding this rather high risk-benefit ratio in advance of initiating such a treatment course is, needless to say, crucial.

Although the BZDs need not be discarded completely as potential agents for use in substance abusers with panic disorder, this drug class remains a treatment of last resort. A maxim to consider is that a substance's abuse potential is directly related to the rapidity of its initial subjective effects on the CNS. Once the drug has reached the nervous system, however, "there are no neuropharmacologic differences among the available benzodiazepines to indicate that any particular benzodiazepine is unique with regard to the risk of abuse" (Shader and Greenblatt 1993, p. 1402).

Where does this leave the clinician who fears giving an addictive agent to a substance abuser? Three considerations may be helpful in determining a treatment plan. First, substance abusers in general prefer to specialize in relatively consistent classes of agents (McLellan and Druley 1977; McLellan et al. 1979) when possible, perhaps because of pharmacogenetic differences between classes of abusers (H. D. Abraham, R. Arora, and J. Crayton, unpublished data, April 1995; Schuckit 1986). This suggests that an individual who abuses cocaine may be less likely than one who abuses diazepam to abuse a prescribed BZD. Indeed, a history of non-BZD abuse is not a strong contraindication to therapeutic BZD use, whereas a history of prior BZD abuse is a virtually absolute contraindication. Second, careful monitoring of prescription dates and numbers will go a long way toward identifying an undisclosed pattern of prescription abuse. Finally, and most importantly, there is no substitute for an ongoing therapeutic relationship sustained with compassion, mutual respect, and frequent clinical reassessments.

Is there a dosage ceiling for the use of BZDs in the treatment of the substance abuser? On the surface, this question may appear to be a thorny one. The clinician's work becomes easier when the aforementioned safeguards remain intact—namely, attentiveness to the details of the pharmacotherapy in the context of a genuine therapeutic alliance. The following clinical vignette illustrates this point:

> Mr. A, a member of a motorcycle gang, consulted a psychiatrist regarding panic symptoms. His job as a carpenter was jeopardized by panic attacks at work. He also suffered severe agoraphobia to the extent that unaccompanied travel from home to work or to medical appointments was difficult. Even when accompanied, Mr. A was unable to separate from his motorcycle. Accordingly, his first interview took place in the outpatient parking lot. During ensuing visits, which included travel alone and graded separation from his motorcycle, it was learned that Mr. A also suffered from post-LSD perceptual disorder and polysubstance abuse without a history of drug dependence. In particular, there was no history of BZD abuse. His social life revolved around his gang. He denied ever having received head injuries, although he had inflicted them. A computed EEG showed spike formation and temporal region irritability. A therapeutic alliance was established around issues of symptom reporting, medication choices, frequency of visits, and graded exposure for agoraphobia. Clonazepam was used over the course of 36 months to a peak daily dose of 12 mg/day. Mr. A was monitored for objective signs of abuse by means of pill counts, physical examinations, and serum drug concentrations. His panic attacks disappeared, and the agoraphobic symptoms declined. His performance at work improved, and prescription abuse was at no point evident. Spontaneously, after 3 years of treatment, Mr. A himself suggested a withdrawal from medication to see if he could remain free of panic attacks.

How long a patient with a history of substance abuse should remain on a potentially addictive treatment regimen for panic disorder is as yet unstudied. Whereas Mr. A's case illustrates the effective use of a BZD in such a patient, one cannot generalize to the class of substance-abusing panic disorder patients as a whole without controlled clinical trials. One viewpoint suggests that when medication helps a patient maintain function and its discontinuation is associated with documented deterioration, prudence dictates a long-term continuation of treatment (Talley 1990). Decisions regarding treatment length are based not on an arbitrarily chosen time interval but rather on the confidence the clinician has in the therapeutic contract, the treatment efficacy, and the patient's reliability.

Chronic Phase

Once an effective and integrated treatment plan has been in progress for a number of months, the focus of treatment shifts to long-term issues related to anxiety and drug use. Therapeutic work is then structured by a mutually chosen strategy. Long-term dependence on drugs, for example, may be interpretable in a psychodynamic therapy as a displacement from earlier objects who failed the patient. Alternatively, self-defeating behaviors may yield to a cognitive or behavioral approach. In being able to generate both drug-like (euphoria) and drug-opposite (withdrawal symptoms) reactions, the stimuli associated with drug seeking and drug taking have been shown to be powerful classical and operant conditioners. Such drug responses have recently been exploited in a behavioral-extinction paradigm to reduce cocaine craving in experimental settings (O'Brien et al. 1992). Compared with control subjects, the behaviorally treated subjects showed statistically superior rates for retention in treatment and for drug-free urines. Vaillant (1992) suggested that parole from prison was one of the more robust predictors of abstinence among heroin abusers. This may be true because prison permits behavioral extinction of drug-conditioned responses—for example, when an addicted person encounters dealers and other addicted individuals in prison who historically served to reinforce drug use, but who no longer can. While the effort to modify conditioned responses in substance abusers is under evaluation, the clinician is well advised to direct the patient's attention to destructive environmental and emotional triggers of drug-using behavior, including triggers of anxiety.

Periodic consultations with the patient's loved ones is advisable, both for external validation and for obtaining new material. One pitfall to avoid is entering into a therapeutic relationship with a substance abuser in which the sole source of clinical information is the patient's own reports. The strong association between substance abuse and antisocial behavior should be kept in mind. Manipulation, misrepresentation, and drug-seeking behaviors will more likely than not outlast the substance abuse for many months, if not years. Clinical decisions must always be made in this light. The following case example illustrates this point:

> Ms. B, a former heroin addict, returned to treatment for anxiety and depression 10 years after a successful detoxification from narcotics. In the interim she had married, borne several children, and gone back to her profession as a musician. At no time during the decade had she returned to narcotic abuse, a point verified by her drug-abstinent husband. Several months previously, however, Ms. B's father had developed a terminal cancer. A physician working in a hospice program, and unaware of his patient's daughter's history, prescribed parenteral narcotics for the father, which he "instructed" Ms. B in administering. As her father lay dying, Ms B administered the narcotics to herself and became readdicted. After her father's death, she was brought back to treatment by feelings of anxiety and suicidal guilt. Ms. B once again achieved sobriety after she relocated with her family to a different state away from known sources of narcotics.

This tragic story illustrates many issues: the semipermanent if not permanent nature of the vulnerability to addiction over a significant span of the patient's lifetime; the necessity of taking a comprehensive family history before prescribing abusable substances; the therapeutic effect of avoiding deeply conditioned drug-using cues in one's environment; and, not least, the addicted individual's capacity to cycle in and out of sobriety, depending on external circumstances and on his or her own commitment to change.

Relapse, unfortunately, is integral to the process of addiction.

Paradoxically, recognition of this fact can free the clinician to work with the addicted patient as a victim of a chronic disease similar to diabetes or schizophrenia. Relapse from abstinence is seldom an indication to terminate a therapeutic relationship, but there may be events in the course of treatment that are. These include a patient's intention, verbally or behaviorally, to continue drug dependence; persistent abuse of prescribed agents; persistent misrepresentation of evidence; failure to fulfill major elements of the therapeutic contract; violence; threats; and similar destructive behaviors. When a legally competent individual chooses to return to a life of drug abuse, the therapist cannot impose a rescue. Other persons close to the individual, however, can use the therapist's help, and tomorrow the patient may be willing to come into treatment once more. If and when that happens, the therapist's door should be open to resume treatment or to assist the patient in finding help elsewhere.

▌ References

Abraham HD: Psychiatric aspects of marijuana, in Psychiatric Medicine Update: Massachusetts General Hospital Reviews for Physicians. Edited by Manschreck TC, Murray GB. New York, Elsevier, 1984, pp 215–229

Abraham HD: Stimulants, panic, and BEAM EEG abnormalities. Am J Psychiatry 146:947–948, 1989

Abraham HD, Duffy FH: Computed EEG abnormalities in panic disorder with and without premorbid drug use. Biol Psychiatry 29:687–690, 1991

American Psychiatric Association: Diagnostic and Statistical Manual of Mental Disorders, 4th Edition. Washington, DC, American Psychiatric Press, 1994

Aronson TA, Craig TJ: Cocaine precipitation of panic disorder. Am J Psychiatry 143:643–645, 1986

Bibb JL, Chambless DL: Alcohol use and abuse among diagnosed agoraphobics. Behav Res Ther 24:45–58, 1986

Bowen RC, Cipywnyk D, D'Arcy C, et al: Alcoholism, anxiety disorders, and agoraphobia. Alcoholism (NY) 8:48–50, 1984

Brantigan CO, Brantigan TA, Joseph N: Effect of beta blockade and beta stimulation on stage fright. Am J Med 72:88–94, 1982

Bromberg W: Marijuana: a psychiatric study. JAMA 113:4–12, 1939

Brown TA, Barlow DH: Comorbidity among anxiety disorders: implications for treatment and DSM-IV. J Consult Clin Psychol 60:835–844, 1992

Cloninger CR: Neurogenetic adaptive mechanisms in alcoholism. Science 236:410–416, 1987

Cloninger CR, Martin RL, Guze SB, et al: Diagnosis and prognosis in schizophrenia. Arch Gen Psychiatry 41:58–70, 1985

Cloninger CR, Martin RL, Guze SB, et al: The empirical structure of psychiatric comorbidity and its theoretical significance, in Comorbidity of Mood and Anxiety Disorders. Edited by Maser JD, Cloninger CR. Washington, DC, American Psychiatric Press, 1990, pp 439–462

Collins GB: Contemporary issues in the treatment of alcohol dependence. Psychiatr Clin North Am 16:33–48, 1993

Cox BJ, Norton GR, Swinson RP, et al: Substance abuse and panic-related anxiety: a critical review. Behav Res Ther 28:385–393, 1990

Craske MG: Cognitive-behavioral treatment of panic, in American Psychiatric Press Review of Psychiatry, Vol 7. Edited by Frances AJ, Hales E. Washington, DC, American Psychiatric Press, 1988, pp 121–137

Dafny N, Gonzalez LP, Altshuler HL: Effects of cocaine on sensory evoked potentials recorded from hypothalamus and limbic structures. Progress in Neuro-Psychopharmacology 3:353–360, 1979

Ellinwood EH Jr, Kilbey MM: Fundamental mechanisms underlying altered behavior following chronic administration of psychomotor stimulants. Biol Psychiatry 15:749–757, 1980

Foa EB, Kozak MJ: Treatment of anxiety disorders: implications for psychopathology, in Anxiety and Anxiety Disorders. Edited by Tuma AH, Maser J. Hillsdale, NJ, Lawrence Erlbaum, 1985, pp 421–452

Fontaine R, Breton G, Dery R, et al: Temporal lobe abnormalities in panic disorder: an MRI study. Biol Psychiatry 27:304–310, 1990

Foy A, March S, Drinkwater V: Use of an objective clinical scale in the assessment and management of alcohol withdrawal in a large general hospital. Alcohol Clin Exp Res 12:360–364, 1988

Galanter M, Peyser HS, Walker RD et al: Position statement on the need for improved training for treatment of patients with combined substance use and other psychiatric disorders. Am J Psychiatry 151:795–796, 1994

Gallant D: Alcohol, in The American Psychiatric Press Textbook of Substance Abuse Treatment. Edited by Galanter M, Kleber HD. Washington, DC, American Psychiatric Press, 1994, pp 67–89

Gerard DL, Saenger G: Out-patient treatment of alcoholism: a study of outcome and its determinants (Brookside Monograph No 4). Toronto, Canada, University of Toronto Press, 1966

Hesselbrock MN, Meyer RE, Keener JJ: Psychopathology in hospitalized alcoholics. Arch Gen Psychiatry 42:1050–1055, 1985

Jaffe JH: Drug addiction and drug abuse, in Goodman and Gilman's The Pharmacological Basis of Therapeutics, 8th Edition. Edited by Gilman A, Rall TW, Nies AS. New York, Pergamon, 1990, pp 522–573

James W: The Varieties of Religious Experience. Cambridge, MA, Harvard University Press, 1985 (Originally published in 1902)

Klein DF, Rabkin JG, Gorman JM: Etiological and pathophysiological inferences from the pharmacological treatment of anxiety, in Anxiety and Anxiety Disorders. Edited by Tuma AH, Maser J. Hillsdale, NJ, Lawrence Erlbaum, 1985, pp 501–532

Kushner MG, Sher KJ, Beitman BD: The relation between alcohol problems and the anxiety disorders. Am J Psychiatry 147:685–695, 1990

Landry MJ, Smith DE, McDuff D, et al: Anxiety and substance use disorders: a primer for primary care physicians. J Am Board Fam Pract 4:47–53, 1991

Leckman JF, Weissman MM, Merikangas KR, et al: Panic disorder and major depression. Arch Gen Psychiatry 40:1055–1060, 1983

Lepine JP, Chignon JM, Teherani M: Suicide attempts in patients with panic disorder. Arch Gen Psychiatry 50:144–149, 1993

Lesse H, Collins JP: Effects of cocaine on propagation of limbic seizure activity. Pharmacol Biochem Behav 11:689–694, 1979

Lesse H, Collins JP: Differential effects of cocaine on limbic excitability. Pharmacol Biochem Behav 13:695–703, 1980

Louie AK, Lannon RA, Ketter TA: Treatment of cocaine-induced panic disorder. Am J Psychiatry 146:40–44, 1989

McLellan AT, Druley KA: Non-random relation between drugs of abuse and psychiatric diagnosis. J Psychiatr Res 13:179–184, 1977

McLellan AT, Woody GE, O'Brien CP: Development of psychiatric illness in drug abusers: possible role of drug preference. N Engl J Med 301:1310–1314, 1979

Meyer RE, Kranzler HR: Alcohol abuse/dependence and comorbid anxiety and depression, in Comorbidity of Mood and Anxiety Disorders. Edited by Maser JD, Cloninger CR. Washington, DC, American Psychiatric Press, 1990, pp 283–292

Miller WR, Hester RK: Inpatient alcohol treatment: who benefits? Am J Psychol 41:794–805, 1986

Mirin SM, Weiss RD, Griffin ML, et al: Psychopathology in drug abusers and their families. Compr Psychiatry 32:36–51, 1991

O'Brien CP, Alterman AI, Walter D, et al: Evaluation of treatment for cocaine dependence, in Problems of Drug Dependence 1989 (NIDA Research Monograph 95). Rockville, MD, National Institute on Drug Abuse, 1989, pp 78–84

O'Brien CP, Childress AR, McLellan AT, et al: A learning model of addiction, in Addictive States. Edited by O'Brien CP, Jaffe JH. New York, Raven, 1992, pp 157–178

Papez J: A proposed mechanism of emotion. Archives of Neurology and Psychchiatry 38:725–743, 1937

Pariente P, Lepine JP, Lellouch J: Self-reported psychotropic drug use and associated factors in a French community sample. Psychol Med 22:181–190, 1992

Pohl R, Balon R, Yeragani VK: More on cocaine and panic disorder (letter). Am J Psychiatry 144:1363, 1987

Regier DA, Farmer ME, Rae DS, et al: Comorbidity of mental disorders with alcohol and other drug abuse. JAMA 264:2511–2518, 1990

Reiman EM, Raichle ME, Butler SK, et al: A focal brain abnormality in panic disorder, a severe form of anxiety. Nature 310:683–685, 1984

Rosenbaum JF: Cocaine and panic disorder (letter). Am J Psychiatry 143:1320, 1986

Sargant W: The treatment of anxiety states and atypical depression by the MAOI drugs. Journal of Neuropsychiatry 3:96–103, 1962

Schuckit MA: Alcoholism and affective disorders: genetic and clinical implications. Am J Psychiatry 143:140–147, 1986

Schuckit MA: Alcohol and alcoholism, in Harrison's Principles of Medicine, 11th Edition. Edited by Braunwald E, Isselbacher KJ, Petersdorf RG, et al. New York, McGraw-Hill, 1987, pp 2106–2110

Schuckit MA, Hesselbrock V: Alcohol dependence and anxiety disorders: what is the relationship? Am J Psychiatry 151:1723–1734, 1994

Shader RI, Greenblatt DJ: Use of benzodiazepines in anxiety disorders. N Engl J Med 328:1398–1405, 1993

Siegel RK: Cocaine: Recreational use and intoxication, in Cocaine: 1977 (NIDA Research Monograph 13). Edited by Petersen RC, Stillman RC. Washington, DC, U.S. Government Printing Office (USGPO 017-024-00592-4), 1977, pp 119–136

Snyder SH: Catecholamines in the brain as mediators of amphetamine psychosis. Arch Gen Psychiatry 27:169–179, 1972

Starcevic V, Uhlenhuth EH, Kellner R, et al: Comorbidity in panic disorder, II: chronology of appearance and pathogenic comorbidity. Psychiatry Res 46:285–293, 1993

Talley JH: But what if a patient gets hooked? Fallacies about long-term use of benzodiazepines. Postgrad Med 87:187–203, 1990

Thomas H: Psychiatric symptoms in cannabis users. Br J Psychiatry 163:141–149, 1993

Thompson JW, Burns BJ, Goldman HH, et al: Initial level of care and clinical status in a managed mental health program. Hosp Community Psychiatry 43:599–603, 1992

Tollefson GD, Lancaster SP, Montague-Clouse J: The association of buspirone and its metabolite 1-pyrimidinyl piperazine in the remission of comorbid anxiety with depressive features and alcohol dependency. Psychopharmacol Bull 27:163–170, 1991

Vaillant GE: The Natural History of Alcoholism. Cambridge, MA, Harvard University Press, 1983

Vaillant GE: Is there a natural history of addiction? in Addictive States. Edited by O'Brien CP, Jaffe JH. New York, Raven, 1992, pp 41–58

Vaillant GE, Clark W, Cyrus C, et al: The natural history of alcoholism: an eight-year follow-up. Am J Med 75:455–466, 1983

Van Ameringen M, Mancini C, Styan G, et al: Relationship of social phobia with other psychiatric illness. J Affect Disord 21:93–99, 1991

Index

*Page numbers in **boldface** type refer to figures or tables.*